Praise for *Mental Illness and Your Town*

"With a father's wit and a reporter's well-honed writing skills, Larry Hayes uses his family's story to offer practical suggestions about how communities can help persons with mental illnesses recover and thrive. This is a wonderful blueprint that spells out ways to change lives and help persons seldom seen or heard."

—Pete Earley, author, *CRAZY: A Father's Search Through America's Mental Health Madness.*

"Larry Hayes—with his background as a journalist, advocate, and parent—understands the challenges that communities face in understanding mental illness. This book outlines the opportunities —and proven steps—we all can take to help 'get this illness out of the shadows and into broad daylight.' Larry helped make my city a much healthier place because of his work on mental illness—his book can help do the same for other communities."

—Paul Helmke, President, *Brady Center/Campaign to Prevent Gun Violence,* Former Mayor of Fort Wayne, IN

"Larry Hayes demonstrates in this book a very rare gift that he has, the ability to reduce complex social problems to simple terms. In addition, he fills the book with practical solutions and ways to reduce the sometimes debilitating effects of mental illness. These will help victims and communities alike to address this reality, that 'We only help a fraction of those who need help.'"

—James C. Howell, Ph.D., juvenile justice researcher

"Like me, Hayes has a history of major depression he has overcome. He is open about this, and about his son's suffering from a major mental health problem. But this is not a 'poor me' story. Rather, it is one of hope and self-empowerment. Hayes is on a mission: to remove the stigma associated with mental disorders, to lead sufferers and their families to self-respect and justice. In these pages, he shows you how you can do the same in your community."

—Bob Rich, PhD., author, *Anger and Anxiety: Be in Charge of Your Emotions and Control Phobias*

In *Mental Illness and Your Town,* Larry Hayes uses his considerable experience as an editorial writer and mental health advocate to show communities what they can do to help the cause of mental illness. Frequently using illustrations from his own experience and his family's experience with mental illness, he gives realistic, substantive and effective examples of what helps and what does not help in a myriad of different areas of society, virtually blasting negative stigma away. The sheer number of good ideas in this document makes it a treasure for any mental health advocate or group. Included is a primer on how to be an effective advocate that is a gem in itself. I can't recommend this book too highly."

—Rev. Barbara F. Meyers, Mental Health Minister, Mission Peak Unitarian Universalist Congregation, Fremont, CA

"Larry Hayes provides families with a real self-help manual that is personal and compassionate, yet practical and hands-on. In my years in the field, I have not seen a book like it. It is long overdue and can only come from someone who has been there—in the trenches. Larry certainly has."

—Stephen C. McCaffrey, President
Mental Health America of Indiana

"I loved reading and learning from this book. I share Larry Hayes' views that we can win the battle against depression, bipolar, and other related disorders if we succeed in counteracting stigma, disseminating knowledge, and enlisting entire communities in the effort. Long ago, I learned that athletes, performers, and everyday citizens who talk about these conditions in matter-of-fact language and with supportive advice become powerful voices in this struggle. Larry Hayes has provided a roadmap as to how to win this struggle. Working together we will do so."

—John F. Greden, M.D.
Upjohn Prof. of Psychiatry and Clinical Neurosciences
Exec. Director, Univ. of Michigan Depression Center

"In *Mental Illness and Your Town*, Larry Hayes has chronicled many great ideas on how communities can improve their systems of mental health care. This enlightening book reflects the 'can do' attitude which Larry has brought to significant challenges and offers strategies on how to move ahead. Several of the ideas in this book have already been implemented in Fort Wayne, thanks in part to Larry's inquisitive and relentless passion to make things better."   —Paul Wilson, CEO
Park Center, the Mental Health Center, Fort Wayne, IN

Mental Illness and Your Town

37 Ways for
Communities
to Help and Heal

Larry Hayes

Library of Congress Cataloging-in-Publication Data

Hayes, Larry, 1938-
  Mental illness and your town : 37 ways for communities to help and heal / Larry Hayes.
       p. cm.
  Includes bibliographical references and index.
  ISBN-13: 978-1-932690-76-7 (trade paper : alk. paper)
  ISBN-10: 1-932690-76-X (trade paper : alk. paper)
  1. Community mental health services--United States. I. Title.
  RA790.6.H39 2009
  362.2'0425--dc22
                                    2008037204

Published by:

Loving Healing Press   www.LovingHealing.com
5145 Pontiac Trail   info@LovingHealing.com
Ann Arbor, MI 48105   Toll Free 888 761 6268
USA   Fax 734 663 6861

*To those who struggle daily
with the challenges of mental illness.*

Contents

Acknowledgement

To friends who helped with research on this book, thanks goes to Terri Milhlbauer, Ph.D., and therapist; John Newbauer, Ed.D, and clinical director of Allen County Juvenile Justice Center; Dr. John Graden, Director of the University of Michigan Depression Center; Andy Wilson, Director of the Carriage House; and Paul Wilson, CEO and President of Park Center.

And to the countless others who have educated and helped me over the years as I explored and advocated for change on a variety of mental health causes.

Also thanks to the Rev. Barbara Meyers who kindly offered suggestions on each chapter and whose help was invaluable.

Many thanks to Evan Davis who pointed me in the direction of this book.

Finally, special thanks and appreciation to my wife and best friend, Toni, for her encouragement, editing and patient support.

About the Cover

On June 20th, 2007, several hundred people from the Fort Wayne community on the Carriage House campus to celebrate the opening of Chad's House, a place for persons from the area to stay when they're training in this highly successful rehabilitation program. Photo provided courtesy of Burke Gallmeister.

Introduction

I should know.

More than twenty years ago, I stood at the bedside of my teenage son as he hovered between life and death in the Parkview Hospital ER. He'd taken an overdose of a powerful antidepressant. Thank goodness he survived. But all his adult life he's battled mental illness. Because of my own experience years ago, I have some idea what he goes through every day.

When John was a small boy, just after my father's death from cancer, I fell into a deep depression myself. I had a six-week stay in the hospital and 12 shock treatments. That time proved to be a hiatus from teaching and family life. It might well have prevented me from taking my own life. Released from the hospital, I joined a therapy group. That helped me reconnect with other people. It was only when I quit teaching school, however, that my depression finally lifted. Through it all, I learned a lot about the shortcomings in a community's response to mental illness. I'm more persuaded than ever that we can do more to help those who suffer find their way back into the mainstream. We can do more to help them find a life of meaning, a life of joy. That's the message of this book for every community.

In 1973, I joined *The Journal Gazette*, Fort Wayne's morning newspaper, to write editorials and columns. I used that platform to advocate on behalf of persons with a mental illness. For background, I drew on my own struggles with depression and my training in abnormal psychology and counseling years before as a divinity student. I interviewed the country's top experts.

I attended conferences. I joined a family support group, a chapter of NAMI, the National Alliance on Mental Illness. State and national advocacy groups honored my writing. I played a role in launching major reforms. I saw our police department adopt a model for intervening when a person with a mental illness got into a crisis. I helped start our county's Suicide Prevention Council. I proposed to the chancellor of Indiana University Purdue University Fort Wayne that he create an institute for behavior studies. That's now a department at the university. I wrote editorials that boosted the opening of the Carriage House, a rehabilitation center modeled after the famous Fountain House in New York City.

So I should know about mental illness. Perhaps the most important thing I know is this. The disability reaches into every neighborhood, every business, every school and more families than you'd imagine. Indeed, our immediate family isn't so exceptional. I just have to go back a generation or two to uncover mental illness on both sides. I've found severe depression, schizophrenia, bipolar disorder, even suicides. Beyond my own family, I've encountered numerous other cases. A former police chief in our city has a mentally ill brother. A judge I know, now in our state appeals court, had a grandmother who had committed suicide. My college roommate's elder son suffers from bipolar disorder. A former secretary of my wife has a mentally ill son.

We tend to think of it as a private, family matter. As a rule, the patient and their families suffer behind closed doors. It's more than that. Mental illness is a serious public health issue. I'm not referring just to the random, inexplicable act of violence that a patient might commit. The disability takes a high toll in lost work time, wages, health care costs and public assistance. Most of all, how we treat persons with a mental illness ultimately stands as a test for how much we care about each other.

Lots of folks don't get the help they need. I've often interviewed agency directors, psychiatrists, psychologists and social workers. I've spoken with family doctors. I'm friends with the parents, the sisters and brothers. Just about all these people often feel frustrated, helpless. They yearn to make a difference.

Here's my answer. Let's take mental illness out of the ERs, out of the psychiatric wards, out of the doctors' offices, out of the group homes, out of the homes of the families whose loved one's mind is out of whack. Let's get this illness out of the shadows and into broad daylight. For the sake of our neighbors, friends, families, co-workers and children, let's engage the entire community.

This book proposes practical ways a community can respond. It's not technical. I leave it to others to decide what all mental and emotional problems to include under "mental illness." I'm excluding no one in your community from playing a helping role. The tragedy that has befallen people with this pernicious condition is not their fault. They're wrestling daily with these demons of their mind. Let's see to it they don't wrestle alone.

First things first.

You should approach the subject of mental illness with a great deal of humility. To treat these various disorders, you are, after all, tinkering with human nature, a matter not to be taken lightly. If the labels have changed through the centuries, the phenomenon has cropped up everywhere. Lincoln's depression was melancholy. Freud's patient suffered from conversion hysteria. In some quarters, people still think the person who suffers is possessed by a demon.

Like the labels, the treatments have varied, from the barbaric that amounted to torture to the benign but useless. If we haven't inflicted physical pain, we've inflicted much emotional distress. We've shunned, isolated and raised false hopes. It's not only those diagnosed with a mental illness who could use fixing. It's the rest of us, too.

I know a lot of families who have changed their ideas, adjusted their lives through struggling with a loved one's illness. They've grown up. They've become more caring, more understanding people. They've come to accept the limits of their ability to fix a child or a spouse. That's humility's reward, a sense of peace with the messiness around you.

But this book isn't about passively accepting the suffering that mental illness brings. It's a busy book, chock full of ideas and proposals and *shoulds*. It aims to challenge people to get busy about the business of seeing to it that those who suffer have a better life. As you dip into this book, checking out one chapter, then another in a different section, please don't think I mean to shame anybody. I mean to get your juices flowing, stir some righteous anger, inspire you with possibilities and, above all, persuade you to lend a hand.

Part I
The Faces

Just as mental illness comes in various diagnoses, it shows up in different kinds of people, at different stages of their lives.

1. Start with Mother and Child

Let me say at the outset that mothers don't cause mental illness. That myth was dispelled long ago. But a mother can foster lifelong mental health. That's tough to do when she's depressed.

In the early months, no doubt Wanda was.

I didn't know it as post-partum depression. Was there such a term in 1965? But I can still see her sad face as I'd walk through the door in our Shirley Place apartment in Cincinnati's western hills. She might still be in her housecoat, strawberry blonde hair not combed. She seemed so frustrated, so inadequate with this baby who had no interest in taking naps during the day. The child seemed happy. The mother wasn't.

I tried to be sympathetic. But in truth, I didn't know how to help her.

Wanda, who died in 1997, was my first wife. We'd been married about three years when Robyn was born, in October, 1965. I had dropped my plan to be a minister and was doing student teaching in the morning and early afternoon, then typing freight bills at Mason-Dixon Truck Lines during the evenings. So the two of them, mother and child, were stuck together for much of the day.

It's pretty common for a new mother to get the blues. Most snap out of it within a few weeks. But for others, the blues turns into a major depression. Untreated the depression can last for years. It can become a lifetime of battling the disability, with only periodic remissions.

The story doesn't end there. Most of us can readily grasp this. The relationship between mother and child is critical to the child's mental health. It's the early bonding. It's the thousand ways a mother communicates to the child that he or she is wanted and loved without condition. Or, in tragic cases, she fails to communicate all that. Maybe the father's love rescues the child, maybe not.

The mother's mental health could be the most precious gift she can give to her child. If you see a baby who appears depressed, listless, it's not a great leap to assume that the mother has been depressed too. She hasn't been able to engage the child.

When the depressed child becomes a toddler, you're apt to find the child cries more easily than other children. That child is the one who develops sleep problems and might act out. In pre-school, that child's problems take on a social nature, disrupting a class and driving the teacher crazy.

As any clinician will tell you, mental health problems in a teenager can often be traced back to early childhood. Fortunately, professionals are beginning to find ways to connect young parents with resources. But reaching everyone who can use the help can be an uphill battle. New mothers may not admit they're depressed. Family members might not pick up on the mother's distress. Or the stigma associated with mental illness blocks out sympathy and understanding.

Outside the family, things aren't much more enlightened. Family doctors aren't well-trained in the pathologies of mental illness. They're especially likely to misdiagnose depression in racial and ethnic minority mothers. Other health care workers face the same limits of knowledge. Further, few persons who work in child care have more than the most cursory understanding of mental illness. As for high-school-age babysitters, I hate to guess. I imagine ignorance abounds.

I'd start with the pediatricians. I don't assume that they're as uninformed as the rest of us. But I'd conduct an inventory on how they deal with a new mother's depression. See if they include any material on postpartum depression in the packet they send the mother home with. Meantime, I'd approach the pediatricians. Find out whether they see any shortcomings in their training and get their proposals for addressing those gaps.

To raise awareness for professionals, we're talking about regular workshops on mental illness. The practices of family doctors and some specialists could be greatly enhanced by adding a psychiatric nurse, psychologist or social worker who is experienced in helping children who suffer a mental illness. As a rule, doctors know that many of the physical complaints people bring to them have an underlying mental health problem. Do most doctors know enough to diagnose a mental illness in the case of an infant or toddler? Do they know enough to treat such a child? These are issues any community's advocates in mental health can investigate.

Short of organizing conferences, advocates can invite doctors to put out reading materials on infant and childhood mental health. They can encourage doctors to run videos on mental health instead of the cable news shows on their TV monitors in the waiting rooms. What about after-school training in mental health for parents? What about offering tips on mental health on the back of menus the schools send home with the kids? And don't assume it's the first time mother who is most at risk. Often, the mother's depression doesn't develop until the third or fourth child. Ask beauty shops to subscribe to parenting magazines. Or barber shops. Be sure to include fathers.

Helping young parents cope pays dividends years into the future. I've interviewed a number of prison officials in charge of young men and women who've become a menace to others. It's as if these officials have memorized some required catechism: "We don't start to fix these people early enough."

Don't misunderstand. Again, I'm not saying that a child's mental health problems can be traced back to a mother's depression. (My daughter, a mother of two teenagers, is a successful teacher and parent.) But even if a child suffers no long-term ill-effects from the mother's depression, the stress on both isn't the best way to begin a lifelong relationship. That stress can only reinforce whatever mischief is in the child's genetic inheritance. Further, let's say the mother got lucky and completely skipped any episode of depression. That fact doesn't completely insulate a young child from a risk of early mental illness.

In recent years, national organizations and a few at the state level have cropped up to offer programs that address mental health in infants and children. Yale's Child Study Center has been a leader. Zero to Three in Washington, D.C., has coached people not to think of the issue in infants and young children as one of a serious mental illness. Most times, we're not even considering medications for treatment anyway. Instead, Zero to Three advises us to think of the issue as one of mental wellness. That's the whole point, isn't it?

Nurture mental wellness in a new mother and she then can nurture it in her child. Mom isn't the culprit. She can be a child's best therapist.

2. Let Them Be Workers

This often is the crown jewel of recovery for persons with a mental illness.

Consider this simple fact. Those who work at least part-time seem do better with their illness than those who don't work. It can beat therapy. It can beat medications. It ranks right up there close to family love. Surveys have found that most people with the disability do want to work. Contrary to the stereotype, about half of these folk actually hold jobs.

I'm most familiar with the clubhouse model. We know it here in Fort Wayne under the name Carriage House. Like nearly 300 worldwide, our clubhouse is modeled after Fountain House in New York City. This is a highly successful pro-work program I'll describe in detail in Chapter 28.

Despite this and other job programs, persons with a mental illness are employed at only two-thirds of the rate of persons in the general population. That figure could be much better. Trouble is, most programs tend to direct people into low-status jobs: dishwashers, custodians, file clerks. Otherwise talented, often highly educated people not only find such jobs boring but also demeaning. Indeed, one thing we've known for years is that persons whose employment is a match for their schooling are more likely to stay on the job and to better manage their illness. Education is the best predictor of success in a job.

Hurdles to greater participation in employment remain. Since some mental disorders strike a person in his or her teens, they often get to middle-age without ever having held a job long enough to develop a work ethic. They don't understand the dos and don'ts. Even at that, a person can start a job, find it stressful and give up within a few days or a week. The person often assumes the illness tripped them up. That's not necessarily the case. Employers, family members and job coaches should encourage the person to stick it out, at least until the disabled person has learned the job. Fact is, you don't have to be mentally ill to find a new job stressful at first. A new job is likely to be stressful for anybody.

Under the Americans with Disabilities Act, a person with a mental illness doesn't have to disclose his or her medical history. Unfortunately, if that person is discriminated against in the workplace, he or she might not know to invoke the ADA, fearing retaliation.

I'd like to see it become routine for local NAMI chapters and other advocacy groups to man a booth at job fairs. It's a good way to offer sound advice to persons with the disability. It's also a good way to make connections with employers and enlighten them about the valuable work a person with the illness can do for them. Advocates, with the support of mental health services, can institute a job fair of their own.

Community leaders always want to see everyone who is capable of working in some kind of a decent job. If you're a NAMI member or an advocate on your own, you can challenge these leaders to survey employers to discover who welcomes those workers battling a mental illness. Meantime, the community mental health center and other agencies can survey those who use their services. Find out who has a job. Find out how long they've been in the job. Find out what schooling they need to get a better job. Join any "Hire the disabled" campaigns. Or let the advocates and agencies launch their own.

I appreciate that a small number of persons with mental illness are too disabled to work. Others will get caught in the trap of having a low, self-defeating opinion of themselves. The idea of a job may scare them to death. But there's a great alternative to a regular job. Persons with a mental disorder can be encouraged to volunteer. That can mean serving at a soup kitchen or tutoring kids in a pre-school. Volunteer work can be just as fulfilling and liberating as working for a paycheck. Volunteering can foster the old-fashioned work ethic and work habits. Volunteer work can be the key to recovery.

A job can be the salvation of most people with a mental illness. I've seen up close the good that having a job can do. It can provide a big boost to a person's *self-respect* so central to recovery. Having a job shows that the person belongs to the mainstream of society and isn't someone merely existing on the fringe. That person is making a contribution. There's something to be said for being able to hold your head high.

3. Save the Suicidal

After my wife Toni and I spent a night in the ER when my son had taken an overdose of a powerful anti-depressant, I was always on the lookout for a way the community could reduce suicide. John's near-successful attempt provided a crash course in the subject.

It was then U.S. Surgeon General David Satcher who gave me the idea for a council.

I called Dr. Phil O'Shaugnessy the afternoon I read about Satcher's call to treat suicide as a pressing public health issue.

I proposed to Phil, an old friend, that he create a suicide prevention council. I didn't have to say much else before he told me to suggest people who should be included on the group.

Phil had served as our coroner or deputy corner for as long as I could remember. Because of that, I was pretty sure he'd been on the scene of more suicides than anyone in the history of Allen County. I couldn't imagine anyone more compassionate with the family, or more helpful.

That phone conversation marked the start of the Allen County Suicide Prevention Council. Sadly, cancer took Phil's life before he could see the fruition of his central role in its creation. We sponsored a major conference featuring *60 Minutes* legend Mike Wallace. Under the leadership of Indiana University Purdue University's Vice Chancellor Kathy O'Connell, we've also put on a number of workshops and training programs. We've hooked up with a statewide suicide prevention network. We now enjoy something of a national reputation. I formally joined the council when I retired from the newspaper.

Our community's suicide rate consistently runs in the mid-range, 10 or 12 a year for every 100,000 citizens. That's the state average and close to the national average. A few states see as few as 6 suicide deaths per

100,000. Several western states can have as many as 22 deaths per 100,000. What's so alarming is that the total suicide rate, from state to state, stays about the same year to year, except that the rate among teenagers and young adults has been on the upswing since the 1990s.

It is interesting to make international comparisons. Russia has a rate three times that of the United States. China's is twice that of our country, as is Japan's suicide rate. But a few countries, such as Sweden and Iceland, which launched a national campaign to reduce suicides, have a much lower rate. In the Philippines and Greece, suicide appears to be extremely rare, although the World Health Organization concedes that some of its figures may not be reliable.

Even if the United States doesn't rank among the worst for suicide, the loss is still staggering. 30,000 or so deaths every year totes up to more than 300,000 deaths over a decade. That's a third more than homicides. As Dr. Satcher put it, this is a major public health issue, ranking right up there with some cancers, and AIDS back in its early years.

To give this a broader perspective, consider that researchers estimate that there are more than 650,000 suicide attempts every year. I assure you, even the attempt by a family member will rattle one's life to the foundations.

Our local council could be a model for any community. It includes doctors, a nurse from the board of health, folks from the hospitals and advocacy agencies, counselors, family members, a survivor of her doctor husband's suicide, an investigator from the coroner's office, an assistant sheriff, a chairperson from the university who also leads the institute for behavior studies and the CEO of the community mental health center. In other words, we've got a cross-section of the stakeholders.

This means that we can get the answers we need to craft any kind of response. How many suicides? Where do we target our efforts? So we begin thinking about who needs to be trained. Persons who work in the jails? In juvenile centers? Nurses and doctors who work in the ER? Family members of persons with a serious mental illness who are most at risk? Family doctors? What about teachers and other school personnel? My answer is yes to all these groups. But you can't just round up the usual suspects in need of education. You've got to get people from these groups interested.

I like the approach where you ask for the advice of somebody who represents the group. Even better: Enlist them to help you plan a training program. The council's main goal is to help people identify suicide risk, and to intervene. That is, we need to intervene in a way that actually prevents suicide.

A small group of community leaders, including the coroner and the head of a mental health advocacy agency, can get things started by looking at the community's resources for suicide prevention. To get you grounded in the issue, I haven't seen anything more comprehensive and practical than the National Strategy for Suicide Prevention, developed in 2000 during Dr. Satcher's tenure as surgeon general. That manual is full of resources. In addition, there are a number of suicide prevention groups that any community council should get acquainted with. There's the National Council on Suicide Prevention, the

American Foundation for Suicide Prevention and the National Organization for People of Color Against Suicide.

It's not easy to show results from these efforts. Suicide occurs episodically. That is, you can go several years and not see a death in the population or demographic group you're following. We have 13 public high schools in our county and several private schools. Some years, none of our high schools will report a suicide. In other years, you'll have two or three suicides. So far, over the last decade, the activity of the suicide prevention council doesn't appear to have affected the numbers. Yet the rate has held steady during a period when the overall population has grown. It may well be that with the relative numbers being so small and the size of the population, less than 300,000, we simply don't have enough suicides to see clear-cut results.

That's been a different story with the U.S. Air Force. When I interviewed the psychiatrist who developed the suicide prevention program for that service, he could say with confidence that by training those in management in mental health and suicide prevention, the Air Force was able to cut its suicide rate by more than 50%, from 15 deaths per 100,000 to six or seven deaths. That's a dramatic drop. Moreover, the population of those wearing an Air Force uniform approaches half a million. The prevention program has worked.

Whether or not we can measure a drop in suicides, the work of the council here remains critical. We are helping to make it OK in our community for people in distress to seek help. We're also giving friends and

family ways to talk to someone who discloses thoughts
of suicide. We're battling the stigma that says we can't
talk about suicide.

I've had teachers, police and friends insist that if
someone is determined to kill themselves, there's
nothing you can do to stop them. I don't believe that.
It's not only that the vast majority of attempts fail. If
you ask anyone who counsels those who are depressed,
you'll hear story after story of suicide prevention. Can
we prevent all suicides? Of course not. But when you
get people to seek treatment for their depression, their
anxiety, their sense of hopelessness, there's a decent
chance they'll find the reason and the strength to live.
They'll find that life is a beautiful thing after all.

4. Rescue Kids in Trouble

"Most kids are here because they pissed off some
adult."

I was doing a phone interview back in the mid-
1990s with the head of the juvenile detention center in
Oklahoma City. It was his opinion that we lock up far
too many kids and don't really protect public safety or
help the kids. Are they bad kids? No. Often they have
major mental health problems. That can lead to
tragedy.

When a 14-year-old girl from Huntington, Indiana,
set fire to the family home and killed her mother and
sister, county officials locked her up in the jail. That
wasn't the half of it. A judge transferred the girl's case
to the adult criminal court. At 14! Then, the state
placed her in the women's prison, the youngest person
ever held there. Somehow, the people who ran the

state's criminal justice system disregarded the history of events leading up to the 1995 fire.

The girl had been abused, physically and sexually. She suffered serious depression. She had been diagnosed with a variety of psychiatric disorders. She had made a suicide gesture at least once. She had been confined for weeks at a psychiatric unit in a Fort Wayne hospital.

To be sure, hers was a major crime. Otherwise, she was typical of many kids who get into trouble and end up in jail. We call it a juvenile detention center. It's a jail. What's worse, in most counties, there's no standardized evaluation of a child when he or she enters the juvenile system. Is the child depressed? Is the child delusional? Suicidal? You wouldn't always know.

The GAINS Center and Mental Health America were able to get a reasonably accurate picture of kids held in 15 counties and nine states. In this survey, researchers found that 70 percent of the kids met at least one criterion for a psychiatric disorder. Further, the survey found that more than 20 percent suffered a disorder sufficiently severe to impair their ability to get through the day.

Let me put that in a national context. James "Buddy" Howell is the former head of research for the U.S. Department of Juvenile Justice and Delinquency Prevention. He points out that our country has 100,000 juveniles locked up in one detention facility or another. That translates into 20,000 mentally ill kids in detention. Since there's no uniform screening in detention centers, who knows what percentage of them even have a credible diagnosis? Who knows how many kids are getting treatment for what surely is a serious mental illness? I've interviewed scores of people who work in juvenile justice. I've served for nearly a decade on the board of the Indiana Juvenile Justice Task Force. The lack of services to mentally ill kids in the system remains the task force's number one issue. If the kids aren't being helped, neither are the families. What a burden that is on parents struggling to understand and nurture a child with a mental illness.

It's no mystery what needs to happen to see that this much-overlooked population of young people gets help. Several national groups, including the U.S. Office of Juvenile Justice and Delinquency Prevention, have offered proposals. And they're backed up with research.

A good place to start is for advocates to find out what if any psychological evaluation is conducted on any kid who gets into the system. You meet with detention officials, any psychologist on the staff and the juvenile judge. Always assume that everyone else is interested in the child's well-being. You can point out that mentally healthy kids usually pose no risk to public safety.

Next, you need to find out whether a kid in trouble gets access to a full range of mental health services. What about the parents? Are they getting help too? You want the parents to be partners in the child's treatment, an often critical missing piece. To get both child and parents the help that they need, you'll want to get the courts to divert the mentally ill child into a center that's less restrictive and that focuses on mental health, not punishment.

Most important, every community needs to enlist the help of advocates, professionals and the media to focus on kids in trouble, especially those with major mental health problems. Wise and humane interventions can make a big difference.

With the support of my newspaper's editorials and legal boost from the American Civil Liberties Union, the Indiana Court of Appeals agreed to move the Huntington girl from the women's prison in Indianapolis to a respected juvenile treatment center in Fort Wayne. There, she received daily therapy and finished high school. At 18, returned to prison, she completed her college degree and has been released. She is now married, has a good job and two daughters.

It's my hope any community would do for every child what people did for this troubled Huntington girl. You never know what child you're going to save.

5. Help College Kids

I guess I had it pretty easy in college.

Part of the reason was that it was a Christian college. I was studying to be a minister, my dream career when I was growing up and into my early 20s.

We had no drugs, no alcohol and little sex I knew of on that 80-acre campus in central Michigan during the late 1950s. Any whiff of cigarettes, sneaked during a hot game of pool at a nearby town on prayer meeting night, brought a stern reprimand from Professor Sears.

But it wasn't just the restrictions that made such a school relatively stress-free. It had to do with the environment of caring and support. Classes were small, and the professors got to know each student. We were a close-knit group. We helped each other throughout romances and our struggles with Greek.

At that time, our students didn't go to therapy, not that some of us wouldn't have benefitted. But, looking back a half-century later, I realize that the place itself was quite therapeutic. I doubt that could be said of any college campus these days, religious or secular.

Any account of campus life today mentions the pervasive stress. In fact, the numbers of college students at risk of suffering a major episode of depression or serious psychiatric disorders has increased dramatically in recent years. When researchers have sampled student bodies, they've found that more than 15 percent of the students exhibit classic symptoms of clinical depression.

In one survey for their Healthy Minds project at the University of Michigan, the researchers discovered that 60 percent of those students suffering from depression hadn't been treated for this quite treatable mental disorder. The staff doesn't see it. The faculty doesn't see it.

No wonder suicide has become the third major cause of death for college students. That's 1,100 lives lost a year on campus to suicide. Who knows how many close calls there are out of the estimated 24,000 attempts?

Naturally, college and university administrators are keenly concerned about students who may become psychotic and take the lives of fellow students. The young Korean student, Seung-Hui Cho, shot to death 32 Virginia Tech students before he turned a gun on himself. This young man not only was mentally ill. He had suffered from the disability since he was in middle-school, if not before. A special judge had ordered him into treatment. No legal authority enforced this order.

It's not that colleges and universities needed such a horrific wake-up call.

Every college and university has counselors and various advisers. If a school gets federal dollars, it's required to offer special help to students with a disability, and that includes those who suffer from a mental illness. National networks have cropped up to address the mental health issues today's college students face. In the spring of 2008, the University of Michigan's Depression Center sponsored a national conference. That meeting drew top experts from campuses throughout the country. Then there's the JED Foundation, with representatives on 750 campuses, which bills itself as the nation's leading organization working to reduce suicide and emotional distress among the six million college students who are served.

But this is a tough challenge. Even if they understand they're depressed, students tend to hide it. They buy into the stigma of mental illness. They're ashamed. Friends advise them to tough it out. If they seek treatment, they fear that would somehow mean losing credits or being forced out of school.

It's not surprising that students would take their prejudices against mental health treatment with them to college. No doubt, their friends sometimes reinforce those attitudes. If the result doesn't end in tragedy, many students still suffer needlessly.

I don't propose that community leaders or mental health advocates butt in. But they have every right to ask questions of university officials.

What mental health services does your college offer students? How do they get access to those services? Are there fees? How are students' privacy rights protected and how are students assured that's the case? How are officials trying to enlighten students about symptoms?

It can also be a matter of life and death for school officials to know when a student such as Cho is under a court order to get treatment. Then what plan do they have in place to see that it happens? An even more tricky issue: Under what circumstances do school authorities notify parents when a student has become mentally ill, and what legal authority do they have to do so?

All you're asking here is for schools to do everything reasonably possible to support and protect the students. Beyond that, it makes sense for community leaders and advocates to offer forums on mental illness for students and faculty.

Our state NAMI enlists persons with the disability to tell their story. It's under this program in Indiana that my son John regularly gives talks to nursing and other students. But the same kind of program could be extended to teach faculty. To be sure, it's helpful for any person in such a position as a professor to learn the facts about mental illness. It can be even more enlightening to get acquainted with someone who manages the illness. That contact can be the greatest stigma buster of all.

Yet another group must be a part of the answer to the stress college students must cope with. I've got the parents in mind. They can join their children during orientation to hear about student services, mental health services included. If they're not doing it now, colleges and universities should offer introductions to college life for parents. And school officials should let parents know what to do if the signs of trouble emerge when the child visits home.

Finally, I believe that, before the children head off in the fall for college, they and their parents need to have conversations about the issue of stress, depression and mental illness. What are the ground rules? When can the parents call? Visit? This is a precious time in a person's life when they're learning to be independent. That development of autonomy is vital to the student's mental health in the long run. But it's just as vital for parents to continue as that family support system the kids always have known.

I wouldn't trade anything for my years in college and graduate school. It's such a time of growth and wonder and maturing. Those years hold such a promise of a happy and fulfilling tomorrow. We need to take every step to see that college fulfills its promise for each student.

6. Reach Out To Soldiers

Most servicemen and women make the adjustment. Too many don't.

Lisa, an old friend of mine, had gone home to Buffalo for the holidays.

She and her sister were having a quiet chat over coffee in the kitchen. Then the world ended.

The shotgun blast from the basement seemed to shake the house.

Lisa's brother-in-law had fought in Vietnam. That was years ago, though.

He was one of those Vietnam vets who never quite found himself. No wounds but lots of scars. It seemed his drinking was the big problem. He'd spend hours at his workshop in the basement, alone, isolated. I'm not sure Lisa even knew that her brother-in-law kept a shotgun in his workshop.

Now we're hearing about the men and women coming home from the wars in Iraq and Afghanistan. I imagine the stories are painfully familiar to Lisa and her sister. At this writing, up to 300,000 servicemen and women suffer from post-traumatic stress disorder. With that catch-all phrase comes a diagnosis of depression and anxiety. That's just part of the story. There has been a rash of suicides. The *New York Times* documented a series of homicides, related to service in the war zone. It's the combat wound that doesn't heal.

In 2008, 1,200 private psychiatrists and therapists nationwide offered to treat these folks free. The idea is to take up the slack. There's a lot of it. The Pentagon only has 1,431 mental health professionals on active duty.

Let's put this in perspective. I'm not counting the guard and reserve of any services.

The Army has 522,000 plus on active duty. The Marines have 184, 000. The Navy has 337,000. And the Air Force has 352,000. Even the Coast Guard (now part of Homeland Security) is a sizable force with more than 39,000 personnel. That adds up to more than 1 million people in uniform. As I said, this doesn't count the guard and the reserve.

Of course, this pales compared to the number of veterans, although they don't necessarily qualify for health benefits. If they do qualify because their illness is service-related, or because of their low income, they likely won't live close to a Veteran's Administration (VA) hospital.

Our hearts go out to those who return from wars wounded in body and mind. Most of us have to believe that the Pentagon and the VA try to do their best to serve the health needs of those who have served their country in this fashion. Then there's the slack.

It may well be greatest when it comes to mental health. Until recently, when a serviceman or woman put in for a promotion, they had to list whether or not they had been treated for some nervous disorder. Defense Secretary Robert Gates concluded that putting that information on the form not only discriminated against those who had been treated for a mental health problem, but also it discouraged them from getting treatment in the first place. That's not right. Gates ordered that question removed from the application for promotion form.

When I was researching how an ombudsman for people with a mental illness might work, the Indiana state-sponsored ombudsman told me she was getting lots of calls from veterans. They didn't want to go through the VA for therapy and psychiatric medications.

This is an issue Congress and the administration need to take up. But in the meantime, communities have plenty they can do to make sure that those on active duty, veterans and their families have full access to mental health services.

The first thing I would do is to investigate what's available in your community.

My city, Fort Wayne, has a VA hospital. It also has a vet center. Both provide some counseling and can make referrals to private counselors.

Next is to place brochures of community mental health services at recruiting stations, VFW and Legion Halls, where veterans gather.

Finally, I believe hosting a conference would provide a great opportunity for people to educate themselves and make connections. A conference on mental health services for persons in the services or veterans and their families could focus public attention on this under-served population. Perhaps such a community-wide focus could even build support for Congress to fill the gaps in mental health services for those who have risked their lives on behalf of their country.

It's commendable that private psychiatrists and therapists have stepped forward to help with the Soldiers Project, the Give an Hour program and the Coming Home Project. But isn't the mental health of our service personnel everybody's business?

7. Get Help to Everyone

The figures give you only a peek at the challenge.

Over a lifetime, one person in 10 will suffer a serious mental illness. But in any given year, one person in four will develop a diagnosable mental disorder.

For the long haul, you've got about 9 percent of the population trying to cope with major depression. (It usually takes months of treatment for somebody to put a clinical depression behind.) Another 2.6 percent suffer from manic-depression or bipolar disorder. About 18 percent cope with serious anxiety. Post-traumatic stress disorder affects a couple of a percent more. Three kids out of 1,000 will be treated for autism. Schizophrenia, the worst mental disorder of all, affects 1 out of 100.

You usually don't count Alzheimer's with these other disabilities. A brain disorder it is for sure. But there just isn't any good treatment and no way to prevent it that we know of now. The Alzheimer's population is 5 million, or about 6 percent and growing, as the baby boomers join the age group most at risk.

If you add the numbers of folk who organize their lives around their various phobias, you're starting to identify the scope of the challenge. What's more, we still lack the all tools to effectively treat the most serious cases of mental illness. Medications don't always work. Talk therapy helps people who have a skilled therapist and the gumption to stick with the therapy.

In the face of such a task, what does a community do? Well, you don't throw up your hands. That's not a moral choice, no matter what tradition of ethics you draw from. More than morality, though, I believe most of us feel it's wrong to let people suffer. We're hard-wired do-gooders, even if we don't always practice what we preach.

One place to start is with a search for people who aren't being served by any agency or support group. You can survey groups at meetings. Would retailers permit people from a mental health association, NAMI group or a community health center to set up a booth on mental health?

I've gone to Walgreen's to get my annual flu shot. I've stopped by a table at our big shopping mall where a nurse from Parkview Hospital took my blood pressure. Mental health advocates committed to reaching out to all populations will find such venues as a drug store or mall once somebody in the group declares we have to do this.

It helps to get the blessing of your mayor and your town or city council. But conducting inventories, not taking names for goodness' sake, can give you a profile of the needs for mental health services. (As a rule, people don't return questionnaires.)

When you inventory nursing homes and agencies that serve the elderly, you're adding another layer of data. What about minority communities? Agencies that serve immigrants and refugees? Mental health advocates can approach the clergy. Even if some clergy don't want to promote any services, most would allow you to place brochures in the church vestibule.

What about the homeless? I've seen estimates that more than half of the folk living on the street suffer from some mental illness. When my wife and I lived in Washington, D.C., I often spoke with them every day on my way to the National Press Building. Washington and other large cities count their homeless in the thousands. Our mid-sized city may have a couple hundred people living in an old car or under a bridge on any given night. Is homelessness inevitable? Or have we dropped the ball?

I suppose if you start sending people who weren't getting served before to a mental health center, you'll find that there aren't enough doctors or therapists to help these folk. But there's a hopeful way to look at this. If you've enlisted more groups into the system, you've automatically increased the numbers and the political power of those who now demand the services.

When you approach state and federal lawmakers, you will have the numbers to make your case for greater funding and an expansion of services. As you demonstrate the need for services, you strengthen the argument for greater support from private foundations. You'll not only have more advocates for better services, but also more success stories.

Mental illness is an awful burden on our society. It's the leading cause of disability, as the numbers I cited earlier demonstrate. But since nobody who suffers is more deserving of help than anyone else, it's imperative for us to reach everyone.

Part II:
The Helpers

One of the great challenges to engage communities in the work of healing is to identify a broad range of resources.

8. Donate Time, Talent, or Treasure

We were drowning.

They sent us Wayne.

He was the guy the Unitarian Universalist headquarters in Boston dispatched to rescue congregations who hadn't figured out how to raise enough money to keep the church humming along.

But Wayne's answer wasn't just about fundraising.

"Challenge members to donate their time, their talent and their treasure."

His reasoning, as I recall, was that you can't get members' invested by appeals for money alone.

"Get members to give of their time and talent, as well as their money. That's the ticket."

Now if there's a better recipe for getting a community to back services for people with a mental illness, I don't know what it would be. Here are 20 ways people can get invested in the cause:

1. Attend meetings. It could be about building a group home in a neighborhood. Show up and assure residents they have nothing to fear.

2. Start fund raisers for mental health programs. In Fort Wayne, a sorority has been raising thousands of dollars each year for the rehabilitation center, the Carriage House. The group invites businesses to create an artistic table display and then hosts a luncheon featuring a dynamic guest speaker. The local NAMI raises money with an annual golf tournament. Meantime, the Carriage House found a big winner with

"Dancing with the Fort Wayne Stars." The "stars" are well-known local people.

3. Put the agencies that help the mentally ill in your will.

4. Volunteer to write grants to foundations that would benefit services.

5. Be a tutor. Lots of people with mental illness had to drop out of school, or were unable to learn while there. In their effort to recover, they study for a GED or enroll in college classes. But their academic skills often are rusty. A tutor can make the difference. And you'll make a friend.

6. Or, help somebody design his or her own college plan or strategy for getting a job. Contact a group home or a drop-in center to offer your help. That could be a donation of your time and talent.

7. Provide respite care. Some sufferers still live at home with family. But giving a parent or sister an afternoon or a weekend to spend by him or herself can help with the family relationships.

8. Set up a foster care program for adults. It's done in Canada. Yes, it would take a great commitment. Often, families become estranged from the disabled person. But having the support of a foster family can help with recovery.

9. Be a coach of a basketball or softball team that welcomes people with mental illness to parti-

cipate. Or start an exercise program at any center that serves the disabled.

10. Be a speech coach. These days, lots of people are out in the community telling their often powerful story of their mental illness. Tips from an outsider can help them be effective.

11. Contribute money regularly to the national organizations such as NAMI or Mental Health America. Check out these and other web sites of other groups to find that group that most clearly fits your interest. (I've added a list of good sites at the end of the book.)

12. Don't forget the local affiliates. Check out the yellow pages and consult web sites. If you like, you can designate United Way gifts to agencies that treat persons with a mental illness.

13. Help with housecleaning. People with a mental illness often struggle to keep up an apartment. With the person's permission, you can schedule a work afternoon every month. It will make the person feel better. And it will help assure that when the Housing Authority comes around to inspect, the apartment will pass inspection.

14. Contribute money for brochures and other literature. Even a small gift can mean that the agency can put out the word on its services and reach more people. If you're artistic, you can help with the design.

15. Make coffee and snacks for meetings.

16. Be a volunteer in something like our mental health community center's Compeer program. In that program, you just spend time and serve as a friend to somebody with a mental illness. The relationship can enrich your life as well as that of the person with mental illness.

17. Train people to answer a suicide hotline. This takes special skill and talent. But you can save lives. What could be more important?

18. Attend workshops on mental illness. Invite friends to join you. Get educated.

19. Call or e-mail your representative or senator to pass laws that give people with mental illness better care and fairer treatment. A few good letters can make a big difference.

20. Join a support group such as NAMI. If none exists in your town, start one.

There's much to be done in the cause of helping sufferers from a mental illness get back into the mainstream. Giving money is only a start. The rewards are greatest when you also give your time and talent.

9. Mend the Net

It's just not right.

We give just enough financial help to people with a mental illness to keep them dependent on government subsidies and frustrated in any attempt they make to join the mainstream.

My son John's situation is typical. His monthly Social Security disability check is less than $600 a month. He's entitled to another $90 in a supplement, known as SSI. Food stamps bring in $55. Medicaid pays for most of the drugs he takes to control his disability, although he still has to spend a few dollars in what amounts to a co-pay.

Even when you add the $200 a month John earns at his part-time job, he's still more than $1,000 a year under the official poverty line for a single person. He's expected to pay a phone bill, gas and electric bills for his apartment and keep his older model Toyota running so he can get to his job. Thank goodness, I'm in a position to help John through the rough spots, with car insurance or a major repair. But he's embarrassed to ask for help, and I'm embarrassed for him. This is not a way to build your self-confidence: asking your dad for money when you're in your late 30s.

Here's what doesn't make sense. Every time John increases his income, he loses a few dollars worth of benefits. His Section VIII housing subsidy drops. His food stamp support drops. He has to pay more for his medications. Yet work is the one thing that can help lift a person with a mental illness out of poverty. It is the one thing that makes him or her feel like a contributing member of society. It is the one thing that allows that person to pay his or her own way in taxes.

Instead of making that path easier, we make it harder, nearly as daunting as dealing with this maddening, crippling illness every day.

It's got to be plenty scary for someone to step out to a well-paying job. Unless it's that special employer who pays health insurance, the person stands to lose Medicaid coverage for expensive medications.

I checked on the price of common anti-psychotic medications with my Wal-Mart pharmacist. Risperdal, often prescribed for schizophrenia, costs over $300 for a month's supply. Lilly's popular Zyprexa, also for schizophrenia, is a whopping $950. Another drug in this category is Clozoril at $367. Tegretol, for bipolar disorder, costs $115 for a month's supply. Depakote, a mood stabilizer, is $211. Antidepressants can run from a few dollars to a couple of hundred.

To live at the edge of poverty creates a lot of stress for anyone. For someone with a mental illness, such stress can only make it harder for the person to get through the day.

I believe that people in any community can make a huge difference, and it shouldn't require turning the world upside down.

Every community should have a clearinghouse where people with mental illness can learn about financial support and guidance. In my city, Fort Wayne, I can count about half dozen agencies that can give a person with mental illness some kind of financial support, from the Fort Wayne Housing Authority to the Wayne Township Trustee's office. Yet there's little contact among them and no coordination, if any. How does one apply for Social Security disability? For Medicaid? What about a housing subsidy? And part-time jobs? And support for those jobs?

A clearinghouse would provide information on all the agencies that offer help, from counseling to case management. It would guide sufferers to food banks, to free health clinics and to groups that have fixed up older cars so somebody could get around a city in which public transportation is lacking. The clearing-house can direct a person to someone to help with per-sonal finances. One agency could loan a social worker to be that contact person for a variety of services. Or several agencies could join to create the clearinghouse.

Connecting people to the resources already in place would be a great start. Because housing is a must, what about launching a Habitat for Humanity with mental illness program? Family members who are retired and others who have carpentry and other building skills could fix up old houses to turn them into group homes, providing your community mental health center can afford to staff more such homes. Social Security and Medicaid won't take housing benefits away if you're getting your housing for next to nothing.

We need to be sure utility companies offer realistic plans so that people can pay their bills and not face the threat of a shutoff of heat or electricity. NAMI families and other advocates shouldn't hesitate to take this cause to utility executives and to the news media.

Surely, we can figure out how to raise Social Security disability and other subsidies so that they provide subsistence at the federal poverty level. That is a minimum step toward fair treatment of this vulnerable population.

What about getting a bank or other financial institution to offer small start-up loans to those with this disability? With the proper medication and other therapy, people can remain stable for years, yes, a lifetime. Mental illness isn't a death sentence. And it doesn't mean that those who suffer can't develop a small business to manage on their own. This is just a thought.

One last challenge: NAMI family members and other advocates for the mentally ill should join the movement for national health insurance. In one stroke, America would instantly wipe out that one great fear for those who are disabled. It would allow more people to test the waters of the working world. National health insurance would add to the long list of millions of tax-paying citizens if more people on disability had jobs.

I believe that communities have a vital role in preventing people with a mental illness from falling through the cracks. We don't want them pushed out on the streets or consigned forever to a life of poverty. It's a matter of humanity. It's a matter of simple justice.

10. Expose the Myths

"Your depression is merely anger turned inward."

The therapist's tone of voice seemed to say, "You poor thing."

Was it true that my depression really was anger? At myself? Well, what was I so angry about? Or was the therapist merely repeating a myth about mental illness? This conversation was way back in 1972. That was long before the theory that fouled-up brain chemistry causes depression came into vogue. Myth or something not quite right, the therapist's remark made me feel that my depression was my darn fault.

Ignorance about mental illness not only makes people feel bad. It also keeps them from seeking and staying in treatment. Even worse, it is the basis for the discrimination that people with this disability face every day. Here are 10 myths I consider the most damaging:

1. Just use your willpower and shake those feelings of depression. That's what Mike Wallace told me his family doctor advised him. Didn't work for this tough, non-nonsense journalist.

Probably won't work for anybody else with a serious problem.

2. Bad parenting causes mental illness. To be sure, when parents abuse a child, that puts the child at greater risk for developing a mental illness later. But good parents can and do have children who develop the disability.

3. Poor life decisions trigger mental illness. Probably not. Your decisions don't have much to do with causing this illness. It's blaming the victim. Of course, telling somebody their decisions caused their illness can make them feel worse.

4. Talk therapy won't help. Not true. In fact, it can help a person overcome major depression. Often, such therapy beats drugs for treating a mild or moderate case. For such major and chronic things as bipolar disorder, it can help the person manage the illness, when used along with the medications. Leading experts I've interviewed advise people with the illness to take medications that seem to help and to find a good therapist too.

5. The illness runs in families. I think this is misleading. Genetics appears to play a role. Studies of identical twins raised apart have found that if one twin develops schizophrenia, the other one has a better than even chance of developing the disability. But this still leaves plenty of room for the influence of life experiences. No matter how

much mental illness can be found in your family, the odds are good that you can avoid it.

6. We know what causes mental illness. Science may be getting close. We know it has a lot to do with both brain chemistry and stress. There's a reason research is ongoing. Remember, we have 100 billion cells in our brains and billions more connections. So, we don't have the final answer, a needle in hundreds of haystacks. My hunch is that we're likely to find it's more than one cause. Children who grew up close to busy streets and highways, exposed to lead before it was banned in gasoline, have been more apt than other kids to get the disability. If a mother gets the flu during pregnancy, research has found her child is at greater risk. I've found studies that cite child abuse and trauma as likely causes. In any case, it bears repeating: Mental illness isn't the person's fault.

7. Mental illness is just another phrase for mental retardation. The two disabilities can be confused, even in a newsroom. It's not uncommon to find people who have both disabilities. But a person with a mental illness can be brilliant or average. Retardation is a permanent condition; the person's intelligence is always well below average. Untreated mental illness in a child or teenager can erode intelligence but not to the degree the person would be considered mentally retarded.

8. Electro-convulsive shock therapy (ECT) is dangerous and should be banned. That's a drastic

and uninformed view. The fact is, it's no more dangerous that any procedure done under anesthetic. It's less dangerous than many surgeries. The common side effect is a temporary memory loss. ECT doesn't always lift the person out of depression. As a rule, it takes multiple treatments. We don't understand why or how it works. But it can turn night into day when nothing else does. I believe ECT may have helped save my life in 1972.

9. People with a mental illness are dangerous. Some advocates claim they're not, almost never. The research says that a person with psychopathology who is also drinking or on street drugs is more apt than most other people to hurt another person. Otherwise, the person with the disability probably is no more dangerous than anybody else.

10. People with a mental illness aren't good workers. This false belief causes untold harm. To be sure, managers might need to make allowances at times, just as they would for any disability. That's federal law, the Americans with Disability Act or ADA. Mental illness is so much more prevalent than we realize. I'm confident there are people in every company, every organization, who battle the disability daily and excel at their jobs. Lincoln and Churchill played their major roles in human history despite their lifelong battle with depression.

I don't claim that I've exhausted the myths. Check out websites of advocacy groups such as NAMI and your local community mental health center. Ask family members and professionals for their list.

Support groups, social agencies and church mental health committees can take on the challenge to expose the ignorance. You can put a simple list in a brochure or, printed in small type, on a business card and on websites. It can be presented as a true or false exercise. Maybe the mythology of mental illness could make a board game.

We've come a long way just in the years since I was hospitalized for depression and felt so ashamed and hopeless. The medications work better, with fewer side effects. Prominent Americans such as Patty Duke, Mike Wallace and many others have told their stories. Still, the myths persist and keep a lot of people from seeking help. They suffer alone, needlessly, in a hell not of their own making. The myths have to go. As they go, so will the stigma. More people will know they don't have to suffer in silence. They'll have the courage to make that appointment with a professional, the appointment that can save their lives.

11. Create Resource Guides

I don't blame Verizon. It's just a phone company. If you don't tell them to add the name of some counseling service, it won't show up in the front of the phone book. That's where they list "Helpful Numbers."

If nobody thought to add the number of the community mental health center on the first page, along with "other important numbers," nobody at Verizon is likely to take it on him or herself to include the center's number.

You're in luck if your problem is drug addiction or domestic abuse. You're in luck if you're trying to find help for your aging mother. Just open the cover of the phonebook and there are the telephone numbers to get you started.

You're going to say that anyone who needs mental health services should simply look in the Yellow Pages. Makes sense. But under what topic do you look?

For "therapists" you've got one listing. It's for the National Board of Cognitive Therapists. Now how would the average mother know she could get help calling this number if her son says he's been hearing voices? In the section on psychologists, you've got PhDs. Our city even has an outfit that advertises "brief therapy."

If you turn to the Yellow Pages for "counseling," then you'll see an array of listings including numbers for Park Center, our community mental health center. The entry lists various services, from addiction services to residential programs. You'll even see a web site.

Under "mental health services," you're faced with a couple of pages, listing therapists, hospitals and coun- seling centers. Such a largely undifferentiated list is what phone companies do with their yellow pages. But we've all had the experience of making several tele- phone calls before you get the right party. (I've had that problem just calling Verizon. Do I want help with the telephone? The TV service? The Internet connection?)

Some years ago, at a NAMI meeting, I proposed that the group develop a community directory on services for people with mental health problems. I even got it started with a couple of others. But one woman stopped coming to the meetings and the other woman ended up devoting more time to her job and her family. She had her priorities straight.

But more than ever, I'm convinced that every community needs to offer more complete help so people can find the services that are right for them. For one thing, the mental health system is fragmented. It's a daunting prospect for an ordinary person to thread through the maze. This is just a hunch. But I suspect that a lot of people just throw up their hands and try to handle mental health problems on their own. Or they attend a session or two with a therapist. Things don't click. They don't search for an alternative. So folks don't get any help whatsoever.

I've got three ways to propose to fill the gap. One would be a comprehensive directory of mental health services. Yes, something like a phone book. The size would depend on how many services your community offers and how much detail you're able to include. Of course, you'd want to list psychiatrists, psychologists and other types of therapists. You'd list the helper's preferred clients, such as family, adolescents, older people perhaps. You'd mention training and length of experience. (Is this a new guy or a veteran with standing?)

If I were organizing such a directory, I'd cross-reference every specialist. So you'd have a listing for psychiatrists. But most of the doctors in that category could also be found under, say, medication management or psychiatric clinic staff. And for all these specialties, do you need a referral? From whom? What about fees? A sliding scale? Do they take Medicare and Medicaid?

The point is to answer questions an ordinary person would consider before ever picking up the phone. People don't seek mental health services when they've got an afternoon to kill on the phone.

As for the agencies, including the mental health centers, the listing should be as comprehensive as possible. Who are the psychiatrists and other specialists on the staff?

Again, what are the fees? How many people receive help every year? You want to make the contact with some confidence that the specialists at the agency know what they're doing.

I intend for anyone with a need or an interest in mental health to have access to such a directory. That would mean placing these books in social agencies, in public libraries, in schools, in churches and in community centers. They could be printed in loose-leaf notebooks to allow for regular updating. A psychiatrist leaves town. An agency moves down the street and changes its phone number.

Who would pay to have such a directory assembled? I think that the agencies and specialists have an interest in getting the word on services out to the community. You start by investigating the cost of collecting the data, the cost of assembling it into a usable handbook and the cost of printing. The cost would vary from one community to the next. And who pays will vary, too. In the end, advocates especially have a vital interest in seeing such a directory created.

My second idea would simply summarize the main directory. I envision a one-pager with a clear title such as "Mental Health Help." These brochures could be placed in grocery stores, pamphlet racks at churches and libraries and businesses. If we're serious about taking mental health issues out of the shadows, we've got to take reminders of the resources and the topic itself out of the Yellow Pages and into the full community.

I mentioned three suggestions. The directory is the first. The one-page brochure is second. The third is to create a website. It's true that the agencies and private providers have their own web sites. How readily can you find them? I propose that the same folks who work in this field and who fight for better mental health care enlist someone to create the omnibus web site. The result would make finding the right mental health services simple and quick. In Fort Wayne, for example, say you don't have internet access at home. You stop by your neighborhood library, plop down at one of the computers and Google "Fort Wayne Mental Health Services." In less than a second, you'd get a list of web sites of all the services in town. And you'd instantly see links to those services including what specialties the doctor or the agency handles, the credentials, fee scale and so forth.

It's inexcusable that we make it so difficult for people to get mental health services. With this crazy-quilt system, communities have only added to the stress and the frustration for sufferers and their families. Access to help should be their last worry, not their first.

12. Enlist Churches

It was her daughter.

She's clean now. Moving back home.

You can almost hear mom's sighs of relief in the back of the congregation.

Every Sunday they line up on both sides of the chalice table to light a candle.

At our church we call it "Joys and Concerns." It's personal.

The joys might seem silly. The Michigan Wolverines beat Ohio State the day before.

It wasn't your particular joy. But it was this alumnus' joy.

But everyone can be touched by the concerns. They express the worries, fears and the hurts of a congregation. People don't say those concerns have something to do with mental health issues. You know better.

I probably stole the idea of starting a mental health committee at the church from somebody. I don't remember who. I thought about it for a long time. Anyway, I enlisted friends in the congregation who have worked in the field for years, got the green light from the minister and the president of the board of trustees.

Our goals are modest. I wanted to introduce the committee to the congregation as professionals who could be a source of information, and help members to make connections with services. Some people might not think to ask the minister first. And in some cases, many members will have long-term friendships with these folk on the committee. No, nobody on the committee will do therapy. My group happens to have no interest in launching a support group, although nobody would object if somebody else started one.

I also felt it would be helpful if people in the congregation knew we had some members who understood the ins-and-outs of mental illness and the community's mental health system: somebody to talk to informally, somebody to give you guidance; somebody who could give you support.

One Sunday in July 2008, the group spoke at the worship hour, each one taking a turn. They told the congregation how they got involved in mental health work. They then spoke of the most important lessons they had learned during all those years in the field.

One church member who does battle mental illness told of the things that worked best for him. My part was to introduce everybody and answer some of the questions people in the audience raised at the end. The service was very well received. My wife Toni also developed a display with a couple of dozen brochures for the fellowship hall.

Around the country, there are experts who help religious leaders figure out how to reach out to people with a mental illness. One person is a Unitarian Universalist minister in Fremont, California, the Rev. Barbara Meyers. She's shared with me a number of ideas that have worked for her. That includes a program developed by Dr. Gunnar Christiansen, another minister. Here, you're advised to start with the church leadership, gaining approval. Then you establish a task force and enlist any pastoral care staff.

This program envisions a support group for clients of mental health services and members of their families. Further, the program suggests you help these clients find suitable housing and even provide jobs. Perhaps most important in this program, the congregation could serve as an advocate on behalf of those with mental disorders to all levels of government.

The point is to get the congregation involved. Let the minister give sermons, perhaps drawing on the great literature of religion. Invite outside speakers who themselves can teach members of the congregation about mental illness and identify the services in the community.

People can't always say why they attend services. But I think most of us are looking for a sense of peace and comfort. Many of us are eager for healing, something that might be missing in our family and work life. Mental health isn't always the language of religion. But the wholeness that's promised is very much a healing of the mind. What more natural place to start the journey than with a group where the goal isn't making money, acquiring material things or fame? Yes, your church, synagogue or mosque can be the place to commence that journey.

13. Open a Suicide Hotline

"If I felt suicidal, I don't know who I'd call." I said.

I guess my mind had wandered. But here we were at our monthly meeting of the Allen County Suicide Prevention Council. For the life of me, I couldn't imagine who to call if I felt suicidal.

At first nobody said a word. Had I just made a totally ignorant observation? Were other people pondering the same thing? Were they thinking about how to kick me off the council?

Then Peggy, our chairperson, said you'd dial First Call for Help.

Somebody else pointed out that that line closes when First Call's office closes, at 5 p.m.

The director of the Mental Health Association said she gets a lot of calls. Her tone of voice told me I should know that.

Then Brad spoke up. He's not only the assistant sheriff. He's a trained Crisis Intervention Team officer. That is, he knows how to help somebody in a mental health crisis.

"Well, Larry, come to think of it, I don't know who I'd call."

Of course, our community has lots of resources. But there's not one suicide hotline, at least not one that everybody knows to call in a crisis and you're not ready to call police.

A few weeks after this council meeting, I brought up the topic with our church's mental health committee. We were sitting in my living room. One of the counselors pulled out his cell phone and dialed the national number. That connected him with one of the 120 regional crisis centers, this one in Indianapolis. In turn, the Indianapolis connection referred us to our community mental health center.

"Well, by now I'm dead," I said at the roundabout, time-consuming telephone call it took us to get to a person. I have no idea how well that person was trained. The national network, of which the Fort Wayne contact was but a tiny branch, refers more than 9,000 calls a month to local centers. Judging from studies, people answering the phones, mostly volunteers, don't always know what they're doing.

When researchers monitored 1400 calls at 14 centers, they found 15 percent of the volunteers failed to meet minimum standards. Often, the volunteer visited for a while, then put the caller on hold. Several got frustrated with the caller and yelled at the person. A few callers already had taken a drug overdose. Yet the volunteer never bothered to ask whether the person was thinking about suicide. In one case I read about, the volunteer asked about suicide but not whether the person had the means. He did and ended the conversation by pulling a string attached to the trigger on a rifle he had rigged.

We don't know if hotlines are actually reducing the suicide rate. It remains as high as ever nationwide, about 30,000 a year. The increase, about 5 percent, is among young people, 10 to 24 years old. Nevertheless, as researchers listened to the hotline calls to the end, they noted the caller sounded less distressed, less hopeless. (It's not the depression alone but the sense of hopelessness that prompts someone to make the attempt.)

Your community should look at the resources for suicide prevention. Is there a hotline? (Federal funds have been available for many centers.) Can everyone readily find out how to reach it? The national number, 1-800-273-TALK, is on the first page of our local Verizon phonebook.

Without a doubt, training is the most critical. Volunteers need to develop considerable skills of empathy. They need to know how to lead a person in distress to work through their problems. These crisis calls are most successful when the volunteers tie empathic listening, sometimes called active listening, to problem solving. Beyond such general approaches, they must feel comfortable asking the person the hard questions directly: Are you thinking about taking your own life? About suicide? (Experts now recommend that you use the word.) Do you now have the means?

Callers often fear that the volunteer will make a record of the caller's telephone number. Keep in mind that some suicidal persons, because of their mental illness, are highly suspicious of others' intentions. But the caller should have a number to reach the same volunteer later. (Who wants to rehash their story to another stranger?) The caller should be told that unless he or she agrees to it or the person seems in imminent danger, a police CIT officer or mental health worker is not going to show up at the caller's door.

Launching a hotline would be a great cause for any NAMI group, a community health center or a hospital. The groups can develop the hotline independently or in cooperation with each other.

One final suggestion: I imagine some people will object to this. But I believe that the hotline should be monitored while always protecting the caller's privacy. This assures that the volunteer phone counselor offers the kind of help somebody in crisis deserves. There's often a chance that the call truly is a matter of life or death.

14. Temper Justice with Mercy

Frank had killed a community activist. She'd let him in her house to get a drink of water after he'd mowed the lawn for her. He'd raped her and slit her throat. He was a scary-looking guy judging from the photographs in the paper taken at his arrest.

I wasn't sure why he'd called me from the jail. To tell his side? I was glad to tell the stories of kids in trouble. But this guy?

We live in such a punitive society. Prison sentences are longer than they need to be. I have to say I don't know what else to do with Frank. He belongs locked up, I suppose for good.

Nevertheless, prison is a terrible place. I've made enough visits at our state institutions to know. If you're not mentally ill when you go in—and 238,000 with a diagnosable psychiatric disorder are in jail or prison on any given day—you're likely to develop depression or anxiety while you're there.

Over the last decade, more than 150 mental health courts have cropped up around the country, from Broward County, Florida, to Cincinnati. Two themes run through these programs. One, they almost always divert only people charged with a misdemeanor. A killer like Frank or a drug dealer wouldn't qualify. Nobody who is deemed a threat to the public safety qualifies. Yet a misdemeanor still can land you in jail. Two, these courts require that the defendant comply with a treatment plan. The judge will assign somebody or an agency to see that the person does follow the plan.

We don't have such a court here in Fort Wayne and Allen County. Marion County, which includes Indianapolis, had a mental health court, although they dropped it a few years ago. But in my county and in others throughout the country, a prosecutor sometimes will transfer a defendant from criminal to civil court. That's when it's clear the defendant suffers from a mental illness. Such a transfer won't happen, of course, if the prosecutor has little understanding of psychiatric disorders.

The benefits of a mental health court look pretty straightforward. The person doesn't go to jail. That in itself can aggravate the illness. Out of jail, his or her treatment with a therapist, therapy group or psychiatrist can continue. If the person's working, that too can continue without interruption. Then there's the savings in tax dollars. It's a lot more expensive to house somebody in the county jail than to provide psychiatric treatment in the community.

These courts are such a recent development that it's hard to be sure that the defendant with a mental illness is better off in the long run than if he or she simply spent a few days in the county jail or was required to do community service. One study of Broward County's experience found good results. There, offenders who'd gone through the mental health court were less likely to commit another offense than those who hadn't been in the program.

A couple of cautions are in order. Some consumers object to the coercive nature of mental health courts. This reminds me of a question I've always had: Can therapy ever be effective if it's not voluntary?

Then you're also creating another court within a local system. For the time being, the U.S. Bureau of Justice Assistance, working with SAMHSA (Substance Abuse and Mental Health Services Administration), provides grant money for these new courts. But who pays when the feds stop picking up the bill?

All that said, it's incumbent on any community to investigate ways to keep people with a mental illness out of jail and out of prison. Mental health courts deserve a close look.

People committing a felony present a greater challenge. Here, as I suggest above, the courts will be looking at public safety as the priority, not the defendant's need for long-term psychiatric treatment. Depending on the charge, a prosecutor can defer prosecution as long as the defendant complies with a variety of requirements: regular drug tests, a strict regimen of medications, meetings with a therapist. If the offender fails to meet one or more of the requirements, the prosecution then can proceed. For such a case, the prosecutor would be weighing the defendant's history, recommendations of therapists and others involved in the person's care as well as on the availability of family support.

You can well object to the coercive nature of this arrangement. But once you've committed a felony, you're bound to face coercion of one sort or another. There's simply no rational way to look at prison time as voluntary therapy.

A prison sentence, however, doesn't have to be the end of the world for someone with a mental illness, or the end of the case. We can provide counseling and other services to mitigate the harm to the victim and to others that a felony has caused. For the offender, we can hold officials in the county and state to high standards of fair and humane treatment of those in their custody. We can insist on competent psychiatric therapy for inmates with a mental illness. We can insist that corrections officers get training in the science and behavior of mental illness. We can insist on greater access for family and friends. Prison officials and guards have much to gain from better treatment of their charges who struggle with mental illness. Above all, we can encourage local agencies and the courts to develop a re-entry plan for the offender. Here, I have in mind not only therapy but work and schooling.

I wouldn't spend a lot of time trying to launch an insanity defense in the case of a major, violent felony. Juries and many judges are suspicious of psychiatric testimony anyway. Such a defense is raw meat for a politically ambitious prosecutor. As for a finding of guilty but mentally ill, a possible verdict in my state of Indiana and in other jurisdictions, the defendant can still end up with a long prison sentence. In one Indiana case I wrote about, a deaf, emotionally disturbed girl set fire to her foster home and killed one other person. Once she completed her prison sentence, she wasn't released on parole but transferred to a state mental hospital. She only thought she was finished with being locked up.

The simple truth is that most offenders eventually get released. They're returned to families, many to jobs and to a productive place in society. Such stories are a constant reminder of why we've got to find ways to help troubled people before their troubled minds set off a series of events that lead to tragedy. When the tragedies do unfold, shaking us to the core, we should do our best to live out those words from St. Matthew (5:7) "Blessed are the merciful for they shall obtain mercy."

Part III
The Personal

Enlisting in the great work of healing doesn't have to be high-minded or motivated by religion of philosophy. Sometimes, it's just everyday stuff.

15. Distribute Self-Tests

I love those things. The self-tests. We've all seen them. Most of us probably have taken them.

"Do you worry too much?"

"How long will you live?"

"Are you eating right?"

No, you wouldn't change your lifestyle on the basis of the results of such self tests.

They're not science. But neither are such tests worthless, merely an entertaining game and nothing more. Many pop up in responsible publications, such as health magazines or journals on child rearing.

Depending on the subject, the tests can tell you something about yourself. They can tell you if you're a worry-wart. They can make you reconsider your high-calorie diet. They can encourage you to reflect on other health habits.

The tests can even prod you into action, say, to see your doctor or spend more time with your children or grandchildren. I think the self tests on depression and bipolar disorder offer a special case.

I say that because so many of us are reluctant to acknowledge we might have a serious mental health problem. We feel anxious a lot of the time. We can't seem to put out the work we used to. We have trouble falling asleep at night. We have trouble getting out of bed in the morning.

Your spouse, son or daughter might not notice that your mood has changed. Most of us have a way of acting cheerful, even when we're down in the dumps. Goodness knows, we'd never seek out a mental health professional for help. We'd need a mighty good reason.

Results of a self-test on depression could give you that reason.

I've seen lots of self-tests in publications on health. But I haven't found a brochure with a self-test that's more comprehensive and user-friendly than the one the University of Michigan's Depression Center puts out. In four, colorful pages, "Beyond Sadness" features faces of people of different ages and ethnic groups with brief statements that offer a crash course on depression. So, just glancing at the brochure, you learn that depression isn't your fault. You learn you don't have to be bawling your eyes out all the time to be depressed. You learn that you can get over it. This stuff is quite treatable.

The centerpiece of the brochure is a checklist of 18 items. Here are a few examples:

"I am often restless and irritable."

"I don't enjoy hobbies, my friends or leisure activities anymore."

"I have nagging aches and pains that do not get better no matter what I do."

"I have trouble concentrating or making simple decisions."

The brochure doesn't claim that if you check any particular number of the items you're clinically depressed. It suggests something more realistic: Take the brochure and the checked items to your doctor. Let him or her advise you on the next step.

The brochure even gives you examples of things you could say to the doctor to open the conversation. It's like having your kindly grandmother take a seat at your side and tell you in a quiet voice that this would be a good time for you to do something for yourself.

I like a couple of other things about this brochure. One is that it lists major organizations and their web sites where you can find out more about depression. In the very back, it cites national medical groups whose experts have reviewed the information in the brochure and found it factual.

Leaders in mental health in your community might want to create a different type of self-test brochure. They'd want to include local resources, including telephone numbers and web sites. Anyone taking on this recommendation should consider a short self-test that can be printed on the health page of the daily newspaper or another local publication. That self-test could also appear on just one side of a brochure that doesn't pretend to be comprehensive like the one that came out of the University of Michigan.

I envision a group of volunteers placing the self-test in doctors' offices, the racks in the vestibules of churches or synagogues, in restaurants, in libraries, schools, in businesses, welfare and Social Security offices and those of other government agencies.

This isn't diagnosis or treatment by a long shot. But well-designed, well-placed brochures with such a self-test can prod some folks who've been suffering to seek help. Indeed, taking the little test can be a first step toward healing. It's a test you can't fail. If you get help, you've earned an A+.

16. Give Them Cell Phones

"Excuse me a minute, Dad."

That's John. He's sitting across from me in our living room. We're in a casual conversation, I suppose about the Cincinnati Reds, or politics. It's no great annoyance that he's interrupted himself to pull his cell phone out of his jeans to look at the phone and see who was calling him or what the text message was.

But that scene, so familiar and unremarkable, gave me an idea. I came to realize that by having the phone on him at all times, John was able to keep in touch with his family and his friends. It was a lifeline in a special way that a cell phone may not be for most of us. Indeed, this everywhere phone represents a kind of therapy; an important adjunct to John's anti-psychotic medications and other boosts to his rehabilitation.

I don't mean to overstate. But no matter how it's done, making connections is important. Let me explain. A person with a mental illness battles a special kind of disability. There's no arm in a sling. No wheelchair. No disfiguring scar on the person's face. The person can seem perfectly normal, if somewhat distracted or without much affect. It's an illness that sits deep inside the person's head. The rest of us can be clueless.

So, the person can feel totally isolated from others, unconnected. You don't belong to anybody. Many years ago, I was there. If anything can reinforce your depression, your sense of hopelessness, it's that feeling of isolation.

Now I don't contend that carrying a cell phone can end that. The illness is too stubborn, too complicated for such an easy fix. But I believe a cell phone can help ease the sense of social isolation.

I asked John if his phone service were only a landline would he use it as much as he uses his cell phone. He chuckled.

"No way."

I doubt if he looks at the cell phone as a vehicle for therapy. But he is connected to other people in ways he never was before.

A cell phone can be expensive. Nevertheless, lots of people on disability already have one. That doesn't mean they're not going without something they need. Many others, however, simply can scrounge up the monthly payment. You can't apply for a contract with some carriers even if you don't have the income to qualify. Or if you get a pay-as-you-go phone, you end up paying double or triple for each minute you're on the phone. If you do get a contract, you may not be able to afford the number of minutes that would allow you to make as many calls as you need to. In any case, the monthly bill can run from $50 to $100 or more, depending on how much it's used.

You'd think all the wireless carriers would offer special rates to people with a handicap. I spoke with Verizon. That company will sell you various packages. But there are no discounts for those with disabilities. By contrast, Centennial offers an $8.25 monthly credit to low-income earners. Further, Centennial takes 50 percent off that company's activation fee.

So this is the story. Some carriers offer special rates, others don't. This presents a challenge to advocates to approach the executives of the wireless carriers and get them to see that it's good business to give people with a disability a break. Meantime, advocacy groups should approach community foundations about funding cell phones for persons with a mental illness.

I see no practical obstacle here. Surely, the technology of this service is such that the cell phone won't be abused. Lost or stolen, an alert to the provider can cut off the cell phone service in a minute. No agency or sponsor needs to get stuck with an outrageous cell phone bill. That brings me to the benefits, which are great.

No matter where a person is, he or she can get in touch with a family member or an understanding friend. In a crisis, the person can call immediately for help. In turn, others can always check in to see how he or she is doing. Or others can just call to ask for a favor. It's not unusual for one of John's friends to call and ask him for a ride, to the supermarket, to visit a mother in the hospital or just to visit.

Sure, the medications and the talk therapy can be important. But nothing is more critical to the recovery of a person with a mental illness than to connect with other people. A cell phone gets the person out of him or herself. Isolation and self-absorption often define the illness. Staying in touch can change all that. This little device can help.

17. Teach the Art of Living

"These are adults, Larry. They don't need classes in how to brush their teeth or make a bed."

Andy is the director of the Fort Wayne clubhouse. He was making the point over a light lunch at Border's that offering classes in life skills to people with a mental illness demeans them and wouldn't work anyway.

I respect the judgment of anyone like Andy who has committed his life to helping people with psychiatric illnesses, and with a respected place in their community. But I've been around people with one form of mental illness or another all of my life. I believe there's a place for good programs that help people succeed in their struggles to recover from mental illness. They deserve no less.

Let's start with job skills. I'm not thinking about teaching anyone how to be a secretary or a custodian or a paralegal. I'm thinking about teaching somebody who may have battled a disability since teen years and has never held a job for more than a few weeks. What should that person know about how to deal with an employer? What should the person know about the importance of showing up on time? About keeping busy? About good grooming? About personal habits? About carrying on e-mail conversations during work hours with friends in Seattle?

You can invite employers to offer classes that cover such topics at group homes, at a clubhouse, at a drop-in center, at your community mental health center. Such an introduction can remove some of the apprehension about work. It's also a good way for employers to get to know applicants as individuals, rather than stereotypes. One more benefit of such a class is that it can allow people to create a mental image of themselves in the workplace. Like an athlete who first creates a mental picture of success before he comes up to bat or starts a race, a person with a mental picture as a worker can also serve as a spur to success.

Getting a person into the mainstream, though, isn't just about the mind. Classes in aerobics have been shown to help people with a mental illness reduce depression, lose weight and develop cardiovascular fitness. In a New Hampshire program called SHAPE, personal trainers work with the disabled to become more physically flexible and overcome a smoking habit. Various programs around the country engage persons with the illness but don't identify them as disabled. They're just another client. Any community can search out resources in that town. What's available? Where would the funds come from? Answer those questions, and then you can team up the trainers in Pilates or Yoga with people, say, who live in a group home or who spend part of their days at a certified clubhouse.

Again and again, such programs have proven that physical fitness has a big payoff in rehabilitation from mental illness. This is no small matter. In fact, physical health comes down to life or death for many. Those who suffer a mental illness have a lifespan that's 10 or 20 years shorter than someone without the illness. You name it. Heart disease, diabetes, cancer all take a heavy toll on people living year after year with the stresses of suffering. The lack of physical activity is just part of it, of course. There's the whole question of diet.

Those who run mental health programs have a responsibility to examine the food they're serving. High on starches? Sweets? Carbs?

What's the portion size? Americans not only eat the wrong things to maintain a decent weight, but also they eat too much. Some antipsychotic medications can frustrate the otherwise reasonable eating habits of even the most dedicated dieter. But where researchers have studied long-term healthy eating programs, they've consistently seen sustained weight loss, less depression and fewer hospitalizations. Workshops on the subject can be the beginning for lots of people.

One last thing. You can't excel in the art of living if you don't have a philosophy of life. Here's where any agency, psychiatric ward or professional offering psychological assistance can play a helpful role. This is not to promote religious beliefs, although that suffices for some people. I'm thinking of how libraries and bookstores have their shelves stacked with books that offer ways anyone can learn to deal with the challenge of living. A therapist can suggest his or her favorite book. Psychiatric wards should vet the books they stock in their libraries. (I trust each one in the country has such a thing as a library.) What about speakers or DVDs on positive thinking? Or, you can invite older citizens who've lived a life for others to meet with consumers and just share their stories. Let such people serve as role models.

I believe that exposing sufferers to various philosophies can help them come to terms with the reality of their illness. That in itself can be healing. Use books, lectures or workshops—whatever prompts reflection, discussion and self-examination. I strongly recommend that everyone write in a journal every day. Any of these things can help people with problems get out of themselves and their often self-absorbed way of looking at the world. If we can teach people the art of living, maybe they won't always feel so left behind.

18. Sponsor Outings

What a good thing any community can do for persons with a mental illness. Getting sufferers out and involved in an activity is one important aid to recovery. Here are 10 examples of what I have in mind.

1. A picnic in the park. This is a low-key activity.
    Nobody who prefers to watch from the sidelines
    is expected to play volleyball. You get your hot-
    dog, slather on the mustard and grab your diet
    Pepsi. If you feel like chatting, you can. Plus, it
    gives you a good dose of sunshine and Vitamin
    D.

2. A trip to the movies. If community advocates are
    savvy, they can round up free tickets from a
    theater and, say, let the folk staying in a group
    home choose what movie they'd like to see. It's
    an outing. It's a social activity. It's another low-
    key thing that strikes a blow against isolation.

3. A long walk. The Carriage House in Fort Wayne
    is directly across the street from Catholic Ceme-
    tery. A psychiatrist who is on our board enlisted
    club members to hike through the grounds.
    Parks will do as well, or any nearby farm in the
    country. Regular walks can take the edge off
    depression. Making it a social event, rather
    than the story of the loneliness of the long-
    distance runner, can nurture the activity as a
    habit. It's a good one, too.

4. Here's another thing to promote mental and
    physical health: Advocates can organize a trip
    to the local Y or other health club. There's lots
    to do in a good facility: swimming, group
    classes, exercise machines, free weights. If
    those who run the place have any sense of
    social responsibility, they'll find a way to give
    your group a discount, or even allow free,
    regular visits.

5. What about visits to museums? A mental illness doesn't interfere with a love of art, science or history.

6. Then there are sports events. The Fort Wayne Wizards baseball team has always offered free tickets for disabled people. What about Little League games? Or high school football and basketball? Watching kids give it their best, cheering for the home team—these get an isolated, lonely person out of him or herself. Attending such games can be yet another low-risk and high benefits outing.

7. I'm thinking of carnivals and fairs, too. You can simply walk around with your friends and look, that's OK. If you're comfortable getting on a roller-coaster, that's OK. You can spend $1 to throw a baseball at bowling pins and hope you win a kewpie doll. You can gather with the farm folk and watch the youngsters parade their prize-winning hogs. Low stress, lots of fun.

8. What about joining a tour of beautiful homes? It might cost a few dollars. But just because someone with a disability couldn't afford a fancy home doesn't mean that person can't appreciate nicely decorated living and dining rooms. Who knows? Maybe this can provide the inspiration to decorate his or her own apartment.

9. Trips to a good library. If you're a mental health worker, or a family member, encourage your client or loved one to get a library card. Just reading magazines or newspapers promises an

enjoyable outlet. No matter who you are, the learning you get from a library visit promotes good mental health.

10. Government meetings. Sure, they can be boring. But any public meeting offers a real world education in how your community is run. If the subject is zoning, taxes or police protection, a town or city council's policies can have an impact on the life of someone who suffers a mental illness.

Such outings, conducted on a regular basis, can help these people to find purpose and enjoyment. Moreover, these examples of outings accomplish one of the most important things you can do to promote recovery and to get those who suffer back into the mainstream of community life.

19. Advise On Estate Planning

Here's a way any support group worthy of the name can make a major difference for those with a psychological disorder.

I'm making a couple of assumptions.

One is that you have a child or spouse with a mental disorder.

Second, your child or spouse now receives or likely will receive government benefits because of this disability.

If it's your local NAMI affiliate, they're likely to invite attorneys who specialize in estate planning to offer a workshop for family members. But a community mental health center or local mental health association can sponsor such a program just as well.

At such a meeting, one thing attorneys are sure to tell you is to have a will and hire an attorney knowledgeable in this field to help you with it.

Don't think of this advice as something that's self-serving. Fact is, laws regarding estate planning vary from one state to another. These laws are subject to change. Further, the Social Security Administration has tightened its rules that govern aid to the handicapped. You probably need a lawyer.

But there's plenty to think about and plenty to learn before you sit down with the legal people.

For example, if your son receives a monthly disability check from Social Security, he won't lose anything from that check from any inheritance. But other benefits can be reduced. The Social Security supplement, SSI, could be lost altogether. Likewise, Medicaid could be cut or also lost. Same is true with food stamps. How much your son or daughter would lose depends on the amount received from these secondary benefits, plus the value of the inheritance.

So if he's permitted to receive $200 a month in SSI and he gets an inheritance at your death of $300 a month, that would wipe out his SSI. Such an inheritance also would translate into a cut in other benefits.

For most people, their property will pass directly to the surviving spouse. That won't be part of any will. Nor will the benefits of any life insurance policy. Those will pass only to the beneficiary named on the policy.

For parents with any assets, I believe the best thing is to create something known as a special needs trust as part of the will.

You specify how much money goes into the trust. But the trustee you designate only distributes the money that your son or daughter needs. For the trustee, also known as the estate manager, you need to choose someone who has a good relationship with your child, someone you know to be sensitive and fair. Some parents already have a pretty good idea of their disabled child's regular expenses and can attach receipts and bills to personal effects to be held by the trustee.

Some families will take a different route. If you have few assets, you can simply identify personal items that would have a sentimental value to your disabled son or daughter. Or you can leave all financial assets to a sibling who is not disabled, with the agreed-upon understanding that the sibling will be fair in distributing assets to the disabled child. Of course, the sibling would be under no legal obligation to share a penny with the disabled child. And the sibling's fortunes may decline to the point that he or she feels they have to tap money that had been set aside for a brother or sister.

What I've offered here is merely an introduction to estate planning. It's a difficult subject that's hard to think and talk about. It can be agonizing enough to worry about your disabled loved one's struggles with mental illness. At least you know you're there to lend support and counsel. Nothing is more important to their well-being than your presence, your love.

But planning for that time when your disabled son or daughter doesn't have your presence can be an act of love as well.

20. Publish Patient Rights

In 1972, I didn't have a clue.

When I checked myself into the psychiatric unit at St. Joseph's Medical Center in Fort Wayne, I didn't know that I had a right to see my psychiatrist's credentials.

I didn't know I had a right to hear about the benefits of the insurance policy the city school district carried on me.

I didn't know I had a right to my records. Or not to be restrained, unless I was likely to hurt myself or somebody else.

I didn't know I had a right to be treated with dignity and respect.

Fact is, I didn't give such things a second thought. I was clinically depressed. I just did what the staff told me to do.

Patient rights can be inconvenient things for providers. In the long run, however, patients understand that they're basically in charge of their treatment, and they're much more likely to cooperate with the psychiatrists and others. They'll be equal members of a team.

A number of states have adopted a bill of rights for psychiatric patients. I especially like the one Arizona developed. It not only sets forth the rights, guaranteeing access to quality care and so forth. In a questionnaire form, it invites patients and former patients to describe any violation of their rights they encountered.

Then there's the "Mental Health Bill of Rights Project," an initiative of professional organizations, including the American Psychiatric Association, the

American Psychological Association and the National Association of Social Workers.

Near the top of this group's list is the right to get all the information you'd care to have about the qualification and experience of the people who are treating you. Under this bill of rights, you have a right to know all about the treatments and what your insurance will cover and what it won't. Once a federal parity law passes, you'll have a right to the same level of insurance coverage as you get for a physical illness or disability. You're promised strict confidentiality.

Every bill of rights I've looked at guarantees treatment no matter your race, ethnic origin, your politics and your ability to pay. In fact, you're guaranteed the best quality of care that's available.

Such issues become critical for the patient when he or she enters a hospital or mental health clinic. Any bill of rights should include the guarantee of a patient advocate. That person wouldn't be a family member or an employee of the institution. Certainly any underage child who comes into the system should automatically be assigned an advocate.

In 1991, the United Nations General Assembly adopted a resolution of principles to protect the rights of persons with mental illness and to improve their care. The resolution covers many of the rights set forth by the professionals' group and by state legislatures such as Arizona's. All address the needs for prompt and professional care of people who have been locked up in prisons or local jails.

As we all know, people who really are political prisoners have been locked up under the pretext that they're psychiatric patients. The former Soviet Union,

North Korea and China are prominent examples. So, under such circumstances, you have no rights, mental illness or not, the U.N. resolution be damned.

Do we honor patients' rights in this country? It's hit and miss. Professionals don't much talk about rights. Yet exceptions exist, in which the adherence to rights is scrupulous. Then, to the everlasting frustration of parents of adult patients, psychiatrists refuse to offer any information about their son or daughter unless they've signed a release. Often the children hate the idea of the parents knowing a thing about their treatment. So they don't sign a release.

I think what hurts the parents so much is that the doctors can be so dismissive that it sounds like the doctor is blaming the parents for their child's disability.

Patient rights are hard to enforce. They feel so inadequate that they are reluctant to challenge anything they're told to do. Meantime, the loved one's illness is such a blow to the family members that they feel powerless.

NAMI and other advocates perform a great service when they educate others about patient rights. But everyone benefits. We're not talking here merely about the legalities or procedures. To broadcast patient rights is to raise the standard for treatment. To broadcast those rights is to hold doctors and other practitioners to quality care for every person.

Just copy the UN resolution. Make lots of copies. Then see that every patient, every family member, every psychiatrist, every therapist, every clinic and every hospital gets one to carry or to post. If we value the patient, we'll honor that person's rights.

21. Heal Families

After one upsetting episode with my son, I asked one of John's psychiatrists what he'd do if John were his son.

"I'd cry," he said.

There was nothing to say after that.

They've yet to figure out a way to let families down gently when they give a son or daughter, spouse, father or mother a diagnosis of mental illness.

Once, in an interview, Rabbi Harold Kushner, whose 13-year-old son died of a rare aging disease, told me that it must be harder to have a son develop a mental illness than to see your son die.

"No closure with mental illness," Kushner explained.

Here's the way it works. You get the diagnosis for your loved one. It's often something worse than you feared. First, you figure you didn't hear the guy right. Slowly, it dawns on you that this probably won't get fixed like a broken leg or a burst appendix. Depending on the diagnosis, this can easily be chronic, even a life sentence. Your loved one gets this scary, mysterious diagnosis and it changes everything in the family.

If you really want to help somebody with a psychiatric disorder, you won't find a better way than to help the families figure out how to cope. I'm not the only father who, quite honestly, knows that in the best of times, he was a mediocre parent. That's when the child is healthy, smart and cooperative. But how do you handle things when your child, as a teen-ager or young adult, hears voices, attempts suicide, drops out of school, closets himself in his room day and night listening to the heavy metal music of Ozzy Osborne?

Lots of people get answers at NAMI. That's the National Alliance on Mental Illness. It's a family support group, some 240,000 people strong. NAMI has chapters in hundreds of cities and towns. Our group meets each Tuesday evening.

I hadn't heard of NAMI until Evelyn Taylor, the local director, showed up at my newspaper office back in the mid-1980s. An earnest, friendly lady, respectful but on a mission, she'd read my editorials on mental illness. I told her about John. She thought she understood what I was dealing with as a parent. Her son was at the state mental hospital in Richmond. Will I come to one of their meetings, at Park Center, our mental health center for northeastern Indiana? Maybe I'd like to write something about her group, too.

That invitation from this angel opened a hundred doors. I thought I knew something about mental health. Hadn't I studied abnormal psychology in the seminary? Didn't the shelves in my study at home hold a raft of books on psychology? Hadn't I fallen into a depression after Dad died? Hadn't I spent weeks on end in a psychiatric ward at St. Joseph Hospital? Hadn't I bounced back, stronger, healthier than ever? When John developed problems, hadn't I dragged him and the rest of the family to a therapist? It turned out what I didn't know would have filled volumes.

I got quite an education in mental illness as I started attending those Tuesday night NAMI meetings. It wasn't just hearing about the advances in the medicines used to treat mental illness. It wasn't just getting the inside dope on the savvy, as well as the

goofy local psychiatrists. It wasn't just finding out
about the shortcomings of services for people with a
psychological disability.

At these meetings, I learned about the struggles of
other families. We'd break into small groups. One was
for parents, one for spouses, one for the sufferers
themselves. We'd tell the stories. Every story was a
heartbreaker. In the parent group, you'd hear how the
son or daughter had just started at Purdue on a full
academic scholarship. She was planning to be a vet or
a dentist. You'd hear about the wedding and the hopes
to move to San Francisco to start a business. You'd
hear about the great job he had just out of high school
as a tool and die maker. I'd tell the others how I was
sure John was headed for Harvard law and a career as
a poverty lawyer. All these dreams. All these hopes.
This illness has entered the family like a home invasion
by masked gunmen. You wonder:

"What's next?"

"When does the other shoe drop?"

You grieve. You grieve because your loved one has
suffered a great loss. You grieve because you have
suffered a loss.

I came to think of the families as heroes. They
certainly became good friends. They've helped me deal
with the guilt and the shame. But we were doing more
than huddling together like cattle in a storm. In sharing
the stories, we were sharing expertise. We were learning
about part-time job opportunities or training for our
sons or daughters. We were learning about the agencies
that helped and about those that didn't. We were
learning how to be advocates for better services, for
fairness in the treatment of health insurance. We were

learning how to adjust our expectations of what the person can do in work, in school, and in family life. We were learning how to cope with our own hurt and fear. We were learning anew to love this son or daughter, husband or wife. What could be more therapeutic, more redemptive than the family's unconditional love and acceptance?

"Pay attention to your own mental health," I told a NAMI conference in Washington one year.

"You can't help your loved one much if you get sick, too."

That's the key.

Of course, NAMI isn't the only way to help families to heal. Other, less formal groups can come together to the same end. Communities should see that any family support group has a place to meet. Foundations can make sure that the group has funds to pay for staff and newsletters. The greater understanding of mental illness throughout the community, the easier it will be for families to seek help. Who are these families?

I've seen estimates that one family in five has a loved one who develops a major mental illness. That's one family on your block. That's somebody you know where you work. That's somebody you see at church.

Some years back, I spoke over the phone with a woman who served then as a state director for NAMI. I suppose I was doing research for tomorrow's editorial.

"I've got four children with a mental illness."

My mouth dropped.

She calmly told me details about each child, every one an adult.

"How in the world do you get out of bed?"

"Well, I love them all."

"Each one is special."

"We just take it a day at a time."

I was ashamed for expecting pity over my own son's illness.

Now there was a hero. Let's heal the families too, I say.

Part IV
The Recruiters

Here's the trick in reaching out to the community.
Don't be shy.

22. Enlist the News Media

I suppose one's first impulse is to call the editor of the paper. But that's not the best place to start.

I always tell people who want their story told to call a reporter.

Here's my reasoning. As a rule, the editors may not know the community very well. Editors spend their days in an office. Their job is to get the most important and interesting stories in the paper or on the air. Unless it's a small newspaper or radio station, the boss doesn't spend his time scaring up scoops on Main Street.

It's the reporters who spend their days in the community and on the phone with the movers, shakers and ordinary people. They're the ones apt to know the person or the organization trying to get news coverage.

Makes sense, doesn't it? Call somebody you know at the paper or the television station.

There's more to it, though. Your immediate goal is to generate interest at the news organization. Say a person with a major mental illness is a champion golfer. He's not ashamed to speak about his condition. It's not the editor who will show up for the men's city tournament. But you can be sure a sports reporter will be there.

In Fort Wayne, Chip Novak is that champion golfer. His mother, Jane, has long been active as a leader in NAMI. It was a natural thing for her to connect Chip with a sports writer. Next thing, a big story showed up on the front section of the sports section, telling of Chip's battle with mental illness.

One thing I like about that story is how it shatters the stereotype of people with any mental disorders. Here's somebody who isn't sitting around all day watching television or otherwise moping about the house muttering to himself. Chip is able to manage his illness by focusing on his drive, his short irons and his putting. He also holds a part-time job.

I don't know if we'll ever banish the stigma of mental illness. But getting stories like Chip's in the paper shows others who suffer that their disability doesn't have to be a sentence of a joyless, meaningless life. Those stories can open the door to treatment and to hope.

At the same time, newspapers or broadcast stations should identify gaps in service and the need for greater financial support. Even the horror stories, which advocates shudder to read, illustrate the problems in services. A Texas woman drowned her five children. But this tragedy followed her premature release from a psychiatric hospital. A New York City man pushed a young woman off a subway platform to her death. He wasn't taking medications that had allowed him to think straight.

The news organization faces a big challenge here. How do you put this story in context? Editors shouldn't want readers to jump to the conclusion that someone with a psychiatric condition is often dangerous. One thing those in a news outlet can do is to solicit comment from local experts. The tragedy offers an occasion to educate people. This is where the advocates come in. Before a person with a mental illness does something terrible, mental health centers, advocates and the psychiatrists need to get to know the reporters and provide contact numbers, day and night. Better still, leaders in mental health would be wise to spend time with the reporters.

It astonished me when somebody who worked in the field would call and ask who they should call about this or that story. After I retired from the paper, I was invited to join the board of the Carriage House, our new rehabilitation center. I believe it was at the first board meeting I attended. A psychiatrist walked in with a check for the center from Lilly Pharmaceutical. He helps the company conduct trials of new anti-psychotic drugs. The check he held up was for $80,000. What an exciting moment for this new center. In 1997, I had managed to get former Vice President Dan Quayle to give a talk at the grand opening. This was a promising start. But a check of this magnitude showed that this was a new institution to be taken seriously. Board President Kathy Bayes passed the check around. We all cheered.

As the only journalist in the group, I suggested we announce the gift to the news media.

"Would they be interested in this as a story?"

I didn't see who asked.

But some board members looked surprised at my suggestion. Warren Sparrow, the director then, nodded.

This is a good rule: Don't judge whether a newspaper, radio or television station would be interested in running your story. Act as though they've been waiting all day for it. Let me add that it can help if you suggest an angle. (The point of the story might not jump out at the reporter or her editor.) The angle I suggested for the Lilly gift was that the Carriage House, the first clubhouse of its kind in the state, has established credibility with one of the country's major drug companies. The amount of the gift wasn't so much the story. It was that Fort Wayne had a new social agency helping people rebuild their lives that was now on the national map.

Some years ago, my newspaper ran a big front page story that announced in the headline that the state-run school for the mentally ill was going to close. There was one little problem. This announcement had nothing to do with persons with a mental illness. It was about the closing of a large institution that cared for people with a developmental disability, mental retardation.

I mentioned the error to a news editor. But he apparently didn't think the distinction important. Of course, it's a big deal to families and advocates. Anyway, we didn't run a correction.

What do you do when a newspaper or broadcast media screws up? If it's a factual error, you should call the news outlet and inform them of it. Sure, you can tell them how stupid they are to get something that important wrong. They'll probably still run the correction. But the next time you call and you only want a clarification to a feature story, you may not find the editor or the writer so accommodating. An approach more likely to win friends and influence people at the paper or the station is to mention at first that you know how hard they try to get things right and to be fair to everyone. That introduction starts you off on the right foot.

One of the best ways of getting the word out about mental illness is by writing letters to the editor or guest columns. I know from research that readers' letters are among the best read features in any newspaper. If you want your letter to be well received and printed in a reasonably short time, make your main point in the first sentence. Keep the letter to 200 to 300 words. No matter how strongly you feel, don't be sarcastic or snotty. That's unless, of course, you want readers to think you're a jerk.

Opposite editorial page pieces require more work and more thought. Length should be reasonable, most such columns in major papers run about 800 words. It's not essential but can be helpful if you're an authority on the subject. You have university degrees. Or you have personal knowledge, experience. If funding of the mental health center has become a public issue, the director is the best person to write the piece. Let's say your community has witnessed a cluster of teen suicides. What does the chairman of a suicide prevention group have to say? What about a column by a professor of social psychology? What could be most powerful in such a painful time would be a column from a fellow student of one of the kids who died by his or her own hand.

As to structure, I appreciated it when somebody called to say they wanted to write an op-ed. piece and did I have any suggestions. Such communication can help you avoid giving the editor too much copy or something too dry to warrant using the space for. But don't fear stating a strong point of view. You're welcome to suggest a headline.

What about convening a news conference? For this you want to write a press release. It needs to be clear, to the point, with contact numbers. And you should see that every media outlet gets it. Then, still ahead of the public event, you call the reporter likely to be assigned to cover the conference. Here, you're making sure somebody didn't pitch your news release in the wastebasket. Let me add a couple more things.

First, it helps to entice a reporter to the news conference if you've got a prominent person to speak at the event. I'm thinking of someone like the mayor, a member of the city or county council, a school board member, the head of the board of health, or the CEO of a corporation. Second, I think you're wise to have several speakers. This gives reporters a variety of people to quote. More quotes mean a longer story, more prominence for your issue.

In more than a quarter century of writing editorials, I was able to keep issues related to mental health and mental illness on the public agenda. Because of my education and my own battle with depression, I took a special interest. I got to know the advocates, the heads of social agencies, and those in the schools who dealt with children's emotional problems.

I was very fortunate to have the backing of the editor and publisher of the paper in my effort to promote the cause. So I would often return to the subject. When people were talking about bringing a clubhouse-type rehabilitation center to the city, I visited the original such center, Fountain House, in New York. I interviewed people involved in the effort in my own city. I wrote about the benefits of a clubhouse and how such a program allowed persons with a mental illness to enjoy work and go to college. I wrote about how transitional jobs helped employers. And in various editorials, I told about the transformation of family life as persons with any serious condition began to find purpose in their lives.

All this editorial advocacy acquainted the community with the clubhouse, which its founders named the Carriage House. Moreover, the new agency gained credibility because the newspaper supported it. That was an enormous plus for supporters when it came to raising money. The family members who visited foundations and businesses would take the editorials with them to show that a clubhouse would be good for the community.

I got creative in one editorial on another issue: mental health parity. The Indiana General Assembly had taken up a bill that addressed the disparity between mental and physical illness in health insurance. Nearly all policies paid much better benefits to treat physical illnesses than for mental illness. So, the lawmakers were being asked to end what advocates regarded as unjust. Business groups, fearing that the bill would increase their health insurance costs, strongly opposed the bill.

My research showed this to be an unwarranted fear. I found that any additional cost would be a fraction of what health insurance costs business. It also made sense that with better health insurance coverage, people suffering from, say, depression would get help earlier and thereby lose fewer working days. In the end, the employer might well save money. Besides, parity is simply an issue of fairness.

Meantime, as I developed my own arguments in favor of the parity bill, advocates established a phone tree throughout the state. NAMI members and others were assigned to contact their local lawmakers to get them to back the bill. I thought of a way to make these contacts more effective.

I constructed a couple of editorials so each argument in favor of parity would be stated in a separate paragraph, identified with bullets. I then instructed the parity leaders to tell the callers to use only one of the arguments, easily picked out of the editorials. I didn't want people to overwhelm the state senator or representative with information. In their enthusiasm, advocates on any issue tend to do that. The bill passed. I was delighted to have played a small part. So news and feature stories aren't the only way you can promote the cause of mental health in a community. Editorials can play a critical role, too. Such efforts can make a big difference in people's lives.

On my bookshelf is *Media Madness*. Written by a psychologist and media critic, Otto F. Wahl, the book cites too many examples to count of how the nation's media have given such a negative image of persons with a mental illness. Wahl's criticism is well deserved. It's little wonder that the stereotype persists. But there's another side to the media and mental illness. I won't speak for the motion picture or television industry. But my experience with newspapers is that people really do try to get their facts straight. They try to make their articles and editorials accurate and fair. After all, this is the standard the industry sets for itself. Moreover, every newsroom has editors, reporters and other writers who struggle with mental health issues themselves or within their own families.

So, enlist the news media. Everyone has a stake in a community's mental health. The media are no exception.

23. Train Activists

If you're going to make change, and goodness knows we need it, you've got to have people who'll write letters to the editor, make calls to legislators and join the public demonstrations for justice.

After all, this is what we're talking about when we're on the hunt for policy change. All these programs, all this research and these therapies can come down to the simple question: What's fair?

It's not fair when most people battling mental illness are forced to live in poverty. It's not fair when they can't find decent housing. It's not fair when they're treated as second-class citizens, made to feel ashamed and unworthy.

But who speaks for those who suffer this disability? The parents, certainly. Many consumers. Applaud their courage. Some professionals. Yes. Supporting them all are the big national advocacy groups such as Mental Health America and NAMI.

All these folk have helped put mental illness on the public agenda. But the stigma persists, a foul odor you can't seem to get rid of. The ignorance. The myths. Despite all the gains, the discrimination persists. At times, it rears its head as downright bigotry.

I suppose most communities have plenty of people who are glad to enlist as activists. They'll give speeches, write letters and make noise. Are they effective?

Sometimes. But they have a greater chance of carrying the day if they know what they're doing. You fight fair. You also fight smart.

In recent years in Indiana, the state NAMI teamed up with a group opposed to the death penalty and other agencies to put forward a bill that would exempt persons with a major mental illness from the death penalty.

I got the ball rolling over a case that involved a young man, Joe Corcoran, diagnosed with paranoid schizophrenia. His crime was huge. Joe had killed his brother and three other guys who were watching a baseball game on TV. His jury recommended the death penalty. The judge ordered it.

My role was to write editorials complaining of the injustice of the sentence for this very sick man. Indiana doesn't execute children or people who are mentally retarded. It shouldn't execute the mentally ill.

In time, the bill to carve out the exemption surely will pass. But some of our advocates haven't always been helpful. In the hallway at the state house, several cornered the chairman of the Senate committee scheduled to hear the bill. He was about to enter the chamber. His committee would be hearing 24 pieces of legislation. Then and there, proponents of the death penalty bill started explaining their bill as lawmakers, reporters and lobbyists passed by.

Needless to say, the senator didn't buy what the proponents wanted him to.

From all accounts, it was a chilly reception. For one thing, these proponents weren't the man's constituents. There simply had been no preparation for this encounter. A chance meeting, it occurred in the wrong place and at the wrong time.

But activists can learn from their mistakes. You've got to figure out how to approach the lawmaker, judge or political leader. Personally, in his or her office? At a public hearing where you offer a formal presentation?

With an avalanche of letters? With newspaper editorials and guest columns?

It's very important for the activist not only to be thoroughly versed in his or her own issue, but also with the group or individual you're targeting to win over. I've found that it's still not a good idea to directly ask for the person's support. There's a better way.

What's worked for me was to attempt to draw that person into your cause. I'll explain what I'm trying to make happen and then ask, "What's your advice on how we can get this changed?"

So you don't start pressing for support. You invite them to join you in some problem solving. My goal here is to get them to take some degree of ownership.

I often will sandwich in an argument or fact into our discussion about strategy. When I was encouraging the city council to adopt a ban on smoking in restaurants, I preferred to talk with each council member privately. If I had written an editorial, I'd ask them what they thought about it. Where did I go wrong? What could have made it more effective?

I tried to keep in mind that the person I was talking to wanted to do the right thing, even if he or she had been a fierce opponent of the smoking ban. For our generally conservative city council, the smokers' rights people and restaurants had a compelling argument: The smoking ban would trample on their freedoms.

My old philosophy professor in the seminary said, "Always make a good case for the other side." Then, personally or in writing, you were to take up the objections of the other side.

Intense speech is a turn off for most people. A quiet appeal to logic works better.

Remember the biblical injunction: "A soft answer turns away wrath." It also helps you get the other side listening.

You want to be sure to enlist a supporter who enjoys a degree of respect and status among those you're trying to persuade to your side. That gives your cause credibility and standing.

You can train activists in workshops. Any group invested in the cause can sponsor the workshop. You want to get speakers who've had success. I'd want a variety of perspectives. So be sure to invite lawmakers, family members and folk with the disability. I'd include a crackerjack salesman or saleswoman who has proven him or herself an effective persuader.

Activists in a community don't need to be pals. But they should form a network.

When a bill relevant to mental health is introduced in the state legislature, you want to convene the activists. You don't want people going off on their own. You don't want five people independently to approach one senate chairperson. Instead, you convene a meeting or two to develop a plan of attack. Then, after that's implemented, you meet again to see what worked and what didn't.

Keep in mind that life isn't going to get better for those who struggle with a mental illness if a community doesn't send forth well-trained activists to be their voice. This is no time for amateur hour. Too much is at stake. For this cause, you want to do everything you can to send in the champs.

24. Observe Special Occasions

Ruth Anne didn't have to remind me.

I knew May was "Mental Health Month."

Nevertheless, the director of the Mental Health Association (known now as Mental Health America) always called to make sure I was planning to write an editorial about mental health that month.

She also would remind me to mention that the association was a United Way Agency. It's any agency's seal of approval.

Such times set aside to call attention to persons with disabilities or to honor secretaries, librarians and so forth give lots of people recognition that's overdue. In the case of mental illness, such occasions, highlighted with nationwide promotions, offer a chance for advocates to educate the public. It gets focused in early fall. That's when we set aside "Mental Illness Awareness Week." So that's twice a year you're apt to see newspaper editorials and TV news features talking about mental health issues.

Every community, though, celebrates special events. One nearby town, situated on the old Erie Canal, celebrates Canal Days. In our part of the country, there are county fairs everywhere throughout the summer. In modern days, it's not just the showings of 4H-raised prize-winning hogs and steers. At one booth, you might find the health commissioner talking about the need for vaccinations or a nurse from the local hospice to explain that service.

In July, our city puts on the "Three Rivers Festival." It's a week of games for kids, a bed race, a raft race on one of our three rivers, an international day that features ethnic foods and dances, an antiques sale, a display of fine art and concerts. To kick off the week is a parade through the city's downtown.

You won't see, however, any float in the parade dedicated to mental health services. NAMI doesn't have a float. The Carriage House doesn't. Or the community mental health center. Such a thing wouldn't be prohibited. Maybe nobody ever thought about creating a float, or at least nobody wanted to put in the time and spend the money to make it happen. Someday, maybe.

Any politician worth his salt knows that any time a big group of people are going to show up, you make an appearance yourself. That's one way you get to be known. The same strategy should apply to anyone with a good cause.

It's impossible to know how much such events help reduce the stigma of mental illness. But every time you get a chance to educate people, you might well have changed a few minds, and, you hope, attitudes.

Our NAMI group here seems to be constantly on the watch for new ways to improve treatment and services for their loved ones who suffer from the disability of a mental illness. They've also found ways to honor those in the community who've been particularly helpful. I recall one banquet in honor of police CIT officers. NAMI played a major role in launching this special cadre of policemen who step in when someone has become psychotic or suicidal. It was a large gathering, over 100 family members, police officials and other guests.

Imagine. We had the police chief and the city's mayor. Our guest speaker that evening was David Kaczynski. It was David who had turned in his brother,

Ted, the infamous Unabomber. David has become a passionate, eloquent advocate on mental illness.

Such events have a way of coming up every year. Well-planned, they attract an audience. Sponsors find it's hard to give up once they've had success.

What about a community forum on mental illness? You invite inspiring speakers and the following year, everybody wants to know when you're sponsoring the event again. One year, I helped bring CBS' Mike Wallace to town for a major address. That, in turn, spurred the suicide prevention group to greater things.

Major public events draw media coverage. They publicize your cause. They let people know about the services. They can remind people of how utterly ordinary, how utterly common, it is for anybody's family to have a member afflicted with mental illness.

These occasions let people talk above a whisper about mental illness. That's what we want. Get this monster out of the shadows. Discover how much a part of the human condition it is. These occasions echo once more the message of hope that anyone touched with one of these disabilities is eager to hear.

25. Enlist State Leaders

Don't leave it to the lobbyists alone.

I'm thinking of the CEOs of the agencies, such as the people who head the state Mental Health America agencies and represent the community mental health centers and the directors of the state NAMI. I'm also thinking of those agencies that represent persons with other disabilities.

They're all indispensable. They know the legislators. They know how to schmooze and when to back off.

They know, or should know, how to get to the point and not waste the time of the state director of the division of mental health or that of a lawmaker. They understand the budget issues. They know what to make a priority and what isn't a realistic goal.

But there's one thing the agency pros aren't likely to do. They usually can't tell their own story.

Who are these people we're trying to help with this bill?

Why can't they make ends meet on the food stamps and the Section VIII housing?

Why do they require such expensive drugs when those so burden Medicaid? Why won't the generics work just as well?

Why shouldn't we make them pay for their petty crimes like everyone else has to?

To engage lawmakers, department heads and governors, you've got to put a human face on mental illness. You've got to help these state leaders feel the human tragedy of mental illness in their own gut.

"They said they never really understood before."

My son John often has mentioned this after giving a talk to university nursing students or students in a sociology class. It's a mission of his to open eyes to what mental illness is all about.

It's the personal touch. It's seeing people up close wounded, often for life, by this disability, not when they're in the depth of depression housed in a psychiatric ward of a hospital. It's hearing about a person's struggle to keep a job, to stay in school, to live independently.

Around election time, the NAMI chapter in Fort Wayne invites candidates to an evening meeting. These days, the meetings are held at the Carriage House, our rehabilitation center. At this evening forum, family members can ask questions and even share personal stories. People with a mental illness are welcome to share concerns about public policy or to share their own story. Of course, the candidates are invited to state their own commitment to improving the life of those who suffer mental illness.

Such a forum has its shortcomings. The first is time. Whether we're facing a city or state election, we're trying to introduce mental health issues to a dozen or so candidates, all within an hour or two. It's tempting for family members to try to extract a campaign promise. That can be awkward. Yet the forum offers the candidate a glimpse of people and issues he or she probably hasn't focused on.

Since the Carriage House opened in 1997, I've taken half a dozen lawmakers for lunch and a tour. I know other board members have done the same. Here, you've got more time to tell the story. The lawmaker can chat with a club member, somebody with a mental illness, and hear that person's story. I believe those visits have won friends for the cause.

People who haven't dealt with a family member who is mentally ill often have strange ideas about mental illness. They can be a little fearful, expecting some irrational outburst maybe. Certainly they're uncomfortable. Such attitudes are no less common among political leaders. This is one reason it's helpful for lawmakers and other officials to meet those who are disabled in different settings. You might want to encourage anybody with a mental illness to enlist in the political campaign of a lawmaker who has been sympathetic to this group of disabled persons. A parent and, say, a daughter with the disability can stop by a lawmaker's office during a session of the legislature.

A less threatening encounter would be through the media. For example, this daughter might write a letter to the editor commending a lawmaker for his or her vote in favor of a more liberal interpretation of Medicaid regulations, explaining how it's helped persons with the disability to manage their limited finances.

What about a campaign contribution? To be sure, people with a mental illness can only rarely afford to give money to a politician. But they could pass the hat and make a big enough contribution to earn an interview with the head of the state senate, or even the governor.

As a journalist, I always found politicians accessible, including those whom I had criticized in editorials or columns. So I suppose my experience doesn't prove that any citizen can get an audience with a lawmaker or other public official. I concede the point. But every politician I've ever known hopes more than to please voters. He or she wants to be liked, respected, loved if at all possible. That means the politician must be accessible. Most of them intend to be. It is, in fact, a prerequisite for getting elected. No piece of information is more important than this if an advocate hopes to see policy turned in the favor of the cause.

You can host banquets, picnics and family outings and invite state and local leaders, inviting them to your home for fund-raisers. You can send them articles, short and to the point, about mental illness and the heroic stories of those who suffer. Sooner or later, mental illness touches each family or a family friend.

It's a reality that must be brought home to state leaders. They've got the power to make a difference.

26. Know Your Meds

It doesn't matter how you get the word out.

Put brochures in the waiting rooms at the doctor's.

Set up a display table of pamphlets in the reading room at your library and station a friendly lady in a business suit there to answer questions.

Make sure the pamphlets list web sites of the major advocacy groups such as NAMI and Mental Health America.

Make sure the pamphlets list the web sites of the drug companies, too.

Or, get your college or mental health center to host a conference or workshop. You can be sure drug companies would dispatch a psychiatrist who conducts clinical trials for them.

Probably nothing in the treatment of persons with mental illness is more misunderstood than the medications. Yet knowing something about drugs offers an insight into the disability you don't get any other way. Ignorance about the medications contributes mightily to the stigma of mental illness.

I'll start here.

Take the most commonly prescribed drug, the anti-depressants. Whether we're talking about the old ones such as Elavil or the newer SSRI's such as Prozac or Zoloft, the idea is to increase the activity of chemicals in the brain that help a person feel reasonably happy. Never mind the technical terms for these chemicals, seratonin, norepinephine and dopamine. Get them to work right and the worst feelings you've ever had in your life melt away.

The fact it often takes such drugs to fix what's gone awry in a person's head tells you it's not a problem you can fix by thinking happy thoughts or by being strong. When I visited with Mike Wallace of CBS' *Sixty Minutes*, he related how his own family doctor reminded him that he was a tough guy and could handle it. Mike's depression didn't lift until he'd been on Zoloft for six weeks.

Let me hasten to add that dealing with medications isn't always so simple. If a person's depression is only moderate, antidepressants often offer little help. Such a person is likely to get over those feelings sooner if they take long, daily walks. And, at least for children and teen-agers, the Food and Drug Administration has determined that some anti-depressants can trigger thoughts of suicide or even suicide itself. Hence the black box on the labels. There's a further caveat: Stopping the medication prematurely.

After White House counselor Vince Foster took his own life, I interviewed the then director of the National Institute of Mental Health, Fred Goodwin. Fred's an internationally recognized expert on depression and bipolar disorder. Yes, he noted, Foster had been on an anti-depressant that his family doctor in Little Rock had prescribed. But after a few months, Fred learned, Foster stopped taking the medication when he felt better. Tragic mistake. Fred said often family doctors will stop the medication before they should. To avoid a relapse, you need to be on the medication at least a year—even if you're feeling better within weeks. Mike Wallace continues to see a psychiatrist "for a tuneup."

And he continues to take his daily dose of Zoloft, this more than 20 years after the onset of his depression.

Each day, the drugs, sometimes called psychotropics, help millions of persons cope. People are able to work at least part-time, go to school, enjoy family and friends and pursue hobbies. In this country, the drugs keep thousands of people out of state mental hospitals. There's a bonus for those who stick with medications that have been working for them. They rarely need to spend any time in psychiatric wards of their local hospital. Now sticking with the medication —that's the trick.

People stop taking the medications for all sorts of reasons. One that most everybody has heard about are the side effects. When I was depressed nearly 40 years ago, the antidepressant I was taking made my mouth feel like cotton. My son John, over more than 20 years, has been on 17 medications that he recalls. Not only did a number of them not work, they made him sicker than before. One gave him a bad case of diarrhea, another triggered panic attacks, still another "turned everything black." In recent years, one anti-psychotic, widely used, tends to cause huge weight gains.

Such unpleasant side-effects help explain why somebody would stop taking the medication. I hasten to add it's not that simple. As John points out, when the person has a bipolar disorder, the manic side can kick in. That produces a feeling of euphoria. "You feel you can do anything," he explains. Persons in this state might well try to do anything. Including throwing away the medications in the honest belief that they've been cured.

There are a couple more reasons that somebody would stop taking the medication or even refuse to take any medication. Their illness has enveloped them in a paranoid world of suspicions and threats. They don't trust anyone, least of all a psychiatrist or family member who wants them to take pills that they're positive are poison. The person rejects the very thing that might spare them the anxiety of the paranoia.

When I was at the paper, I covered the case of Joe Corcoran who had shot and killed four men, including his older brother Jim. The men were watching a ball game in the sister's home downstairs. Joe had been napping upstairs. Later, he told the police in a taped interview that he thought Jim and the others "were talking about him." His paranoid schizophrenia was only diagnosed after his trial. At the county jail, and later in the state prison, Joe calmly related to me how the CIA had been sending him messages through his teeth and how cellmates could hear him confess to "sexual secrets" in his sleep. I don't believe Joe, now on death row, ever believed he was mentally ill.

Such denial isn't uncommon. I've talked to a researcher who theorizes that some mechanism in the brain chemistry blocks any belief that the person might be mentally ill. Given how vehemently some people resist the diagnosis, this theory makes sense to me.

John has observed that it's not only the general public who see persons with a mental illness as a stereotype and stigmatize them. Even those who suffer buy into the stigma. With the stigma comes a great deal of shame and self-loathing. Why take a medication that seems to confirm such a negative view of oneself?

The stigma stands in the way of treatment. No wonder most people with a diagnosable mental illness don't seek out a psychiatrist first. Like Mike Wallace, they take their complaints of mental distress to the family doctor, who may or may not know much about the right medications or the nature of the illness.

We've all read the news accounts. A man in New York, with a history of mental illness, stops taking the medications that have been keeping him sane. At an impulse, he shoves a young woman off the subway platform to her death into the path of a subway train. In Texas, a mother of five, recently released from a psychiatric hospital, drowns her children. And at Virginia Tech, a disturbed college student, diagnosed as paranoid but not taking any anti-psychotic drug, kills 31 fellow students before killing himself.

Could these tragedies have been averted? If these persons had taken the right anti-depressant or anti-psychotic drug, would that have spared the lives of their victims?

I wouldn't be dogmatic about it. But medications just might have made the life-saving difference.

It's hardly true that people who don't take medications for mental illness are dangerous. The cases I cited are the rare and tragic exception. Untreated, however, the illness robs a person of his or her dignity, of the ability to do a job, to excel at school, to form good relationships with other people. Untreated mental illness isolates and demeans a person. It robs him or her of a place in the community's mainstream. It robs a person of hope.

To be sure, the meds aren't the whole answer to mental illness. Sometimes they're useless. So far, not one of them has been developed that will cure one darn thing. But for many people these drugs represent a giant leap forward to rehabilitation. Let's get that story out. And let's get it straight.

27. Monitor Commitments

We got lucky with Judge David Avery.

In our county, he oversees all commitments of persons whose illness has made them a danger to themselves or others. He's been doing it now for some years. Further, he belongs to several mental health committees in the community.

He goes to the Suicide Prevention Council meetings, attends and gives reports for the community group that helps plan training for the police department's Crisis Intervention Team. He serves as one of three chairs for the county mental health coordinating council, which brings together all the stakeholders.

Here's a judge who's involved. He knows family members. He's friendly with persons who suffer from a mental disorder. He knows how the various agencies are supposed to work. It has all afforded him a broad perspective on the problems of those with a mental illness, and on the players in the community.

So what do you want if your loved one has become dangerous or gravely disabled and therefore meets the state standard for an involuntarily commitment? What do you want to happen if your loved one has a real shot at recovery? What do you want to do to make sure this person is treated humanely and with justice? The answer to all this is simple. You want a judge who has insight into the illness and compassion toward those who suffer.

To me, an involuntary commitment of any duration is a last resort. You're depriving a person of his or her basic civil rights, guaranteed in the U.S. Constitution. That person often doesn't understand the proceedings, or opposes them. My heart sinks when I hear of someone I know who's being considered for a commitment. At the same time, the person's disability may be so grave that such a commitment is the only thing that can save the person. If realistic alternatives existed, I'd shout them from the rooftops.

So advocates must get involved in order to develop better ways of dealing with this serious problem. It doesn't matter if we're talking a short-term commitment in a local hospital or long-term in a state-run facility. Start with the judge. Schedule a meeting with that person and hear about his or her policies, get his thinking. If you spot shortcomings, state your concerns.

If an attorney is up for an appointment by your governor or is a candidate in an election for judge, you need to get acquainted. If you like how this person thinks and what he or she says, you need to back that person's elevation to the court. If you don't like how this person stacks up, you need to be vocal in opposition.

The role of the judge in the success or failure of an involuntary commitment is simply too critical to take whatever the state or county's political system produces. Beyond meeting, and hearing about policies, the advocates should encourage the judge to visit group homes, tour the state hospitals and your hospital psychiatric units.

You want to know, further, who is keeping track of the commitments. How long are patients kept at the state hospital? Every state sets limits. What are they? What's the follow-up when people are released? When it's a 72-hour involuntary commitment, do most of the patients choose to stay in the hospital for more treatment? Who makes sure the person continues to receive the proper care when they're out of the hospital? A stay in an institution isn't likely to be of any lasting benefit without good after care.

Sad to say, but at least a half of those committed to a state institution find themselves returned under a court order in less than a year. Of course, relapse varies from state to state. To be sure, the newer medications have improved the relapse rate somewhat. Even at that, once a person is released, it may not be easy to keep him or her compliant with the medication. I imagine most if not all people who are committed regard it as a person setback, a failure.

In each state, you can assume a public defender or private attorney will represent the person who is being evaluated for any long-term involuntary commitment. This is another key figure in the proceedings. Does that lawyer have an understanding of mental illness? Does this person seem uncomfortable attempting to communicate with the patient? The public defender assigned to these cases should have had a lot of experience with the patients and with families. You want to be sure the judge has confidence that this is the right person handling these cases.

Judge Avery has started to conduct commitment hearings through closed-circuit television. This means that the patient doesn't physically appear in a courtroom but in a more comfortable setting at the local hospital, reducing the stress on both the patient and on family members.

Some experts prefer an outpatient commitment option. Here, the judge is likely to set strict requirements the patient must adhere to. The patient must follow the drug regimen, and respect any curfew the family or group home sets. He or she must report regularly to a therapist and back to the court. The outpatient commitment gets mixed reviews from people I've interviewed. Success depends largely on the quality of the services that surround the person. Of course, some people are simply too sick and disabled for them to function outside an institution.

But here's another place where advocates have a role. They need to inquire of the judge how he determines whether a patient is a suitable candidate for an outpatient commitment. What services will the person receive? What will it take for that person to comply with the court order? Full cooperation can mean a more lasting recovery. A successful out-patient commitment saves tax dollars, too.

Those of us who advocate for persons with a mental illness would prefer not to think about involuntary commitments. Locking people up, however benign its purpose, rubs many of us the wrong way. The limited success of such commitments reminds us of how our knowledge of mental illness is so rudimentary. The lack of great results shows how inadequate our treatments remain for so many who suffer. But care we do. Get involved we must.

Part V
The Innovations

Want to put your community on the map when it comes to mental health? Launch new programs.

28. Establish a Clubhouse

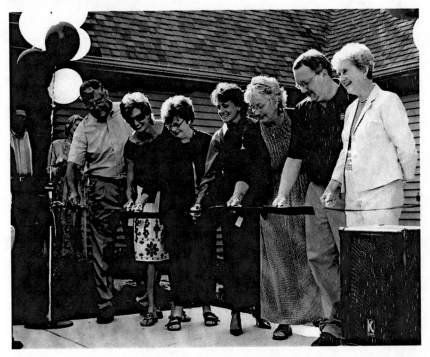

Author's son John joins celebrities in the ribbon cutting ceremony for Chad's House.

They are (left-to-right): Dr. Steve Glock, whose late son Chad was a Carriage House member; Dr. Glock's daughter Brenda Gerber; Joyce Glock; Tina Nomarry, president of the Pi chapter of the sorority that raised funds for Chad's House; Susan Simpson, national president of Psi Iota Xi; John Hayes and Patsy Dumas, president of the Carriage House.

Photo provided courtesy of Burke Gallmeister.

More information about Carriage House is available online at www.fortwayneclubhouse.org.

"Even when you're gone, Dad, I'll always have the clubhouse."

It's impossible to overstate how much good this rehabilitation center on the city's near-north side has done for my son John over the past decade.

I recall driving one foggy morning to the Fort Wayne clubhouse, which for years housed doctors' offices, and turning into the driveway as the fog started to lift. On the hill to my left, this old, white mansion silently arose from the mist as if by magic.

Our clubhouse is like nothing else. Here they attempt to restore the broken hearts and lost souls who have been the victims of a mental illness. It doesn't resemble any hospital's psychiatric ward. It's no group home. It's no private sanitarium where patients roam from one garden to another. It's not a drop-in center where you play ping-pong or thumb through an outdated magazine. The people who go to the clubhouse aren't patients or "consumers." In fact, it was ex-patients from state hospitals who established the first clubhouse, Fountain House on West 47th Street in New York City. This was back in the 1940s. It wasn't a place for sick people. It was established for those who were determined to get their lives back.

Fort Wayne's first clubhouse director was an Australian, Warren Sparrow. He often said, "We leave the illness at the door." Now they're just club members. To be sure, the staff of social workers helps supervise activities. But they don't require any club member to lift a finger. You're a club member. So you're a free agent. You make your own decisions. You're treated as an equal, not some subordinate who has to kowtow to the director and his staff.

As a rule, club members show up and expect to work where they're needed. They can be preparing the low-cost lunch, taking orders, serving, helping with the clean-up. Or the club member might be heading out of the building for a part-time job at a library, a law office or a restaurant.

These jobs, known as transitional employment, put the club member on the first step to regular work. For its part, the staff does everything to make sure the member succeeds on this first step.

It works this way. Even before the club member is assigned to this job somebody on the staff goes through the training for it. Then the club member learns what's expected, at first with the staff member at his or her side. If the club member can't go to work that day, the staff member fills in. What a bargain for the employer. The work will always get done.

Back at the clubhouse, things can get intense and personal. You might see a club member tutoring somebody who is preparing to take his GED that afternoon. Or somebody else might just be listening as a friend pours out his heart over some personal problem.

What I'm describing is a small, close-knit community, more like a family. The Fort Wayne clubhouse has been the home-away-from-home for more than 800 club members, with 250 coming on a regular basis. Those preparing the meals can count on 60 hungry folk sitting down for what probably will be the best meal of the day. Club members keep track of others. They phone and send cards to those who are sick or who are having a birthday. And they keep track of who's coming and who's going.

We call our clubhouse the Carriage House, for good reason. When the NAMI families, led by Dr. Steve Glock and his wife Joyce, acquired the property, a rickety old carriage house stood at the back of the five-acre property. Just as the buildings needed rehabilitation, so do the club members strive to rehabilitate themselves every day they show up.

I'm aware that other such programs have come along for those who suffer a mental illness. One, known as PACT or ACT, offers wrap-around services of nurses, case managers and doctors to help people get on their feet and stay there. PACT places people into jobs, makes sure they're stable and helps keep them out of the hospital. It's a good program. By comparison, a certified clubhouse sees that the club member stays on the job a bit longer and enjoys greater job satisfaction. That's the research. No wonder the clubhouse model has grown into a worldwide movement with more than 300 programs, from Denmark to Japan to Australia. There are over 200 in the United States alone. They're not all in cities, either. A number thrive in small communities. To be certified, they must adhere to the clubhouse standards, developed by the International Center for Clubhouse Development in New York City.

The Fort Wayne clubhouse operates in partnership with Park Center, this area's community mental health center. Park Center pays for the Carriage House staff and is reimbursed by Medicaid. But the clubhouse does its own hiring and firing. Club members have a say in every one of those decisions. Other clubhouses survive as independent social agencies. But each one must raise funds to continue operating.

My son can talk all day about the near miraculous change in the lives of his friends at the clubhouse. When one man started coming, he just stood in the corner by himself. Finally, people coaxed him to join in. He started attending club meetings. In no time, it seemed, he was manning the snack bar. Another man didn't speak to anyone when he first came. In a few years, he was singing at the clubhouse annual talent show. He's even been able to hold part-time jobs.

For this dad, the clubhouse has been his son's salvation. It's more than a place to go. It's a place where he's found his self-confidence, his self-respect. He hasn't felt the need to go to the hospital in years. He's found a mission in life. He's developed into a spokesperson on mental illness. He gives talks at colleges and to civic groups. The International Center for Clubhouse Development in New York put him on its faculty. In no time, the ICCD was sending him around the country to visit and help certify other clubhouses. It's my most earnest wish that every community would develop a place like our Carriage House where people like John could learn to put their God-given talents to use, where they could find themselves and learn to live with hope.

For starters, check out the web site of the International Center for Clubhouse Development (ICCD.org), and the web site for Fountain House in New York: (Fountainhouse.org.) You're then just a click away from a revolution.

29. Open a Depression Center

Depression.

You don't have to explain what it is.

I've seen it in faces.

I've seen it long ago in my son's face as he sat across from me at Hall's restaurant wolfing down his cheeseburger and onion rings. He was just a teenager then, but with the movements of an elderly person.

No expression. He looks at his plate. He only raises his head when he senses I'm staring at him.

I've seen it in my wife Toni's face, a quarter of a century ago. She's in her upstairs study at our old house. She's supposed to be writing her dissertation. But the page stays blank. She's sitting on the register with a blanket around her to keep warm. She has no expression, either.

I've seen it on other faces, those of fellow workers. If you ask, they'll just say they're having a rough day. It also was in the faces of people in psychiatric wards, when I visited my son John during his 12 hospital stays. And in 1972, I saw it when I looked in the mirror: Depression.

I only learned about community depression centers a few years ago. That's when I read Andrew Solomon's op-ed piece in *The New York Times*. Solomon's book about his own battle with depression, *The Noonday Demon: An Atlas of Depression*, won the National Book Award. His NYT column appeared just months after the University of Michigan opened the country's first Comprehensive Depression Center in Ann Arbor and after he attended their board meeting, and participated in a discussion about establishing a national network of depression centers analogous to the network funded by the National Cancer Institute.

Just the name of this center takes mental illness out of the shadows. When I visited the center, Dr. John

Greden, a psychiatrist, told me that donors feared the name would turn away patients. He stuck to his guns. Depression center it is. It's a giant leap for mankind, I say. Think of the titles we give other agencies that treat mental illness. If we don't call them something like "Menninger Clinic" or "McLean Hospital," we just give them a one-word name, such as "Lindenview," which in Fort Wayne has become Park Center's transitional program. (Park Center is the area's community mental health center.) Now it's true that such institutions can treat, train or conduct research to help people who aren't, strictly speaking, mentally ill. But mostly, they do deal with this population. Why not say so in naming the institution? We know one big reason. It's the stigma.

Because of the stigma many people take their mental troubles to the family doctor first. Because of the stigma so many take their troubles no further.

The new center at the University of Michigan is about a lot more than attacking the stigma with a title. The colorful decor, the sunny, open atrium, the light-filled spaces throughout and the impressionistic art in the offices and the halls create a feeling of hope. That's the message of everyone you talk to at the center: Depression is treatable.

This illness messes up the lives of 19 million Americans every year. That translates into 30,000 suicides and an untold number of attempts. When coupled with bipolar disorder, it's the number one cause of disability worldwide. The sum is an Everest of misery. I've been there. You feel it as a huge weight that puts you into slow motion. You can feel it as a knot that extends from your stomach to your throat. If you can even make it out of bed and get to work, you can't concentrate. You're ready for bed after you've gulped down supper. That is, if you felt like eating.

A depressed child is a lonely child. He can be an angry child who won't cooperate with parents or teachers. Schoolwork suffers. He gets no joy playing games. If such a child has friends, they would be few indeed. Cartoons on TV fail to amuse. The child's depression becomes the family's daily burden.

When I was depressed, I was impossible to live with. My first wife, Wanda, pleaded with me not to be so nasty toward my two children. I dreaded heading off for the high school where I taught. Most of the time I felt too lousy to think about suicide. I never admitted to anyone I was depressed or might have considered killing myself.

With all this in mind, given the numbers of people afflicted, a center for the study and treatment of depression promises a degree of hope that seems positively revolutionary.

The University of Michigan Depression Center sets the standards for such institutions necessarily based at large universities attached to teaching and research hospitals. Representatives of a number of universities across the country have attended forums in Ann Arbor with the intent of creating such a center in their own region. In early 2008, the second depression center opened at the University of Colorado in Denver.

Since learning of the University of Michigan center, reading about the program and talking with people there, I've been in awe at the depth and breadth of what they're doing. That center boasts some 180 staff, including psychiatrists, social workers and therapists.

Naturally, the annual budget runs into the millions of dollars. The center houses the largest data bank in the country of DNA from victims of depression or bipolar disorder and their families, as well as for people with no history of these disorders.

You can be treated for depression or bipolar disorder at the center. You can learn about the research, the treatments and the ways to support persons at any one of the center's seminars and workshops. You can tap into their web site to administer your own screen for depression. Or, in that region of the country, you can invite one of the specialists listed on their speakers' bureau roster to talk at a conference on depression.

Just as not every city or major medical center houses a cancer center, not every city or major medical center has the ability to house a depression center. That's not the gist of this proposal. When I visited the University of Michigan Depression Center, Dr. Greden told me of his vision for satellite depression centers. These satellites wouldn't offer everything that's at the main center. But they could tap into the parent institution's speakers, data bank and workshops. The satellite might send its psychiatrists and therapists to the main center for training. Further, the satellite might refer patients or take referrals. On an informal scale, even a small town hospital might name its psychiatric ward the depression center and make treatment of depression and other mood disorders its focus.

Getting mental illness out of the shadows is the point. Any community that wants to take that step should make the journey to Ann Arbor, Denver or any city where there's a movement to create a depression center. The visit would be inspiring. It would give far-away community leaders ways of adapting the programs and services of the major center to their own town or city. I believe any community can tie together the services that already are in place to create a depression center.

We don't have all the answers. We don't fully understand the brain chemistry that's involved in depression. Or why a loss in one person's life sends him or her spiraling downward in despondency while the next person copes with the same kind of loss. Medications seem to help many people. Talk therapy can be the salvation for others. Just getting your mind off yourself, through exercise or helping someone else, can lift your despair. But none of these solve this great mystery of the human condition. I'm hoping that a network of depression centers and their satellites countrywide will someday shed even more light on that mystery, even unravel it. Then we'll wonder where the sad faces have gone.

30. Call the C.I.T.

I couldn't believe how quickly they showed up.

We had called 911 after our teenage son, just released from a psychiatric hospital, had gone on a rampage through the house. We had no clue how to settle him down.

It's scary to call the police in such an emergency. You don't know how an officer will handle a family crisis. They're trained to take control. To accomplish that, some officers don't hesitate to get rough, sometimes with tragic results. As a journalist I had too frequent occasions to write about such outcomes.

In our family's crisis, this might well have turned into a tragedy. The officers at our home believed my son when he told them he'd flushed a bottle of anti-depressants down the toilet. It wasn't until the officers got him back to the psychiatric hospital that it was clear he had misled the officers. An hour or so later, an ER doctor explained that our son was lucky. He had swallowed the bottle of anti-depressants. If the psych-iatric hospital staff hadn't gotten him to the ER, he probably would have died.

For years, the episode haunted me. I wondered if the police had been better trained they might not have taken my son's word about what had happened to the anti-depressants and gotten him to the ER sooner. The more I looked into the matter, the more I realized that the police training in handling a mental health crisis had shortcomings.

Back then, officers got only a few hours of training by the mental health association and a cursory idea of the services. That training focused on the officer's role in getting somebody who was out of control into the hospital for an involuntary 72-hour commitment. They had little instruction on the variety of mental illnesses. They didn't learn how to de-escalate a crisis. They didn't spend any time getting to know people who suffered from a chronic mental illness. The call to hospitalize the person came by telephone. No profess-ional saw the patient face-to-face to assess what should happen. The assessment usually was made on a family member's say-so. This meant lots of folk who didn't need to be hospitalized ended up in the hospital. Worse, because the officers had little training, they sometimes escalated the crisis, rather than defused it. Officers and patients got injured.

Over a period of twenty years, we saw a couple of tragedies. Officers, not understanding the psychological dynamics involved, and believing they were threatened, shot the person in crisis to death.

The Memphis model helped put a stop to such needless tragedies in our city.

I was at a NAMI conference in Washington, D.C., when I attended one workshop about the revolutionary way Memphis police handled a mental health crisis. In 1985 a Memphis police officer shot to death a person with schizophrenia. Leaders of the local NAMI chapter protested. Memphis police Maj. Sam Cochran and Dr. Randy DuPont, a psychologist, developed a 40-hour program to train an elite group of officers. By the time I'd heard about Memphis, Cochran and DuPont had trained officers from Albuquerque, N.M., and Portland, Ore.

When I got back to Fort Wayne from the conference, I met with then Mayor Paul Helmke to tell him about Memphis. I just told him a few things. I didn't overwhelm him with details. I stressed the benefits to the community. In turn, Mayor Helmke assembled a committee of mental health experts. While that committee didn't complete the job, a new mayor, Graham Richard, dispatched several city officers to Memphis. I joined them for an orientation. I spent one night riding with one of the CIT officers. Then I saw how skillfully he'd learned to deal with a person who had a mental illness. I was sure that almost any officer could be trained to do as well.

When I returned to Fort Wayne, I gave Mayor Richard a copy of news stories about the Memphis program. Because he so quickly grasped the benefits, I wasn't surprised when he gave his complete blessing to the creation of a CIT program for Fort Wayne police. I backed up my private urgings with editorials.

Only a year or so later, we had a community oversight group and were interviewing candidates for the Fort Wayne CIT team. The training came next. Psychiatrists, social workers, hospital personnel, even those with a mental illness put the first group of about 50 officers through the paces over several days of intensive training. Today, 10 years later, Fort Wayne boasts more than 150 trained CIT officers. The Memphis model represents a revolution in how police here treat persons in a mental health crisis.

From January through April, 2008, a typical period, CIT officers responded to over 300 such calls. And over 290 persons agreed voluntarily to be taken to the hospital. There were no 72-hour involuntary detentions. Twenty people were stabilized at the scene. There were no deaths, even though, according to the police report, "the party was armed" in 30 situations. There was only one arrest. That last fact in itself illustrates the transformation. Years before CIT, scores of persons during a comparable period would have been taken to the county lock-up to be jailed. What's more, the training has created a corps of officers who treat disabled people with respect. You no longer hear of police referring to them as "mentals."

Research on how CIT works in Memphis revealed similar results. Plus, the researchers noted that under this program, officer injuries have been down.

I'm sure that CIT police training could be improved. Indeed, I continue to be impressed with the high caliber of people who join the team. But I think it would be great if officers in training spent more time with anybody who is mentally ill but not in a crisis. That exposure can help further dispel the stigma the officers associate with mental illness. The Memphis officer I rode with got to be friends with a number of persons with a mental disorder. I recall that we stopped by two apartments just to check on somebody. After a brief visit, we were on our way.

Over the past few years, Fort Wayne has become a training center for area CIT officers and we've helped spread the word about the change in police relations with those suffering mental illness. Major Cochran now calls us the flagship CIT city, testimony to our success in confronting what can be one of the most troubling things for people with a mental illness and their families. Every community has an obligation to see that some police officers will answer the emergency call not to subdue the bad guys but to rescue a sick person in trouble.

31. Get an Ombudsman

Who speaks for the person with a mental illness?

An ombudsman could be one good answer.

I can appreciate what such a role can mean as well as anyone. As the longtime editorial page editor of the morning paper in Fort Wayne, I routinely got an earful of people with a complaint.

"It's a waste of time talking to you!"

"Transfer my call to your circulation department!"

"I'm canceling the paper!"

Such conversations didn't end well, whether or not I had anything to do with the person's letter being cut. Usually that would have been somebody with the thankless job of copy editor. But the person doing the complaining was mad at me. I was that idiot.

How often I wished I could have turned the complainant over to the paper's ombudsman. Alas, we employed no such person.

Two of the country's major papers, *The New York Times* and *The Washington Post,* do employ a person who, if not called an ombudsman, performs this as a service for readers. Both papers allow the ombudsman to operate with a high degree of independence. That consumer advocate even writes a newspaper column about the paper's screw-ups.

"The customer is always right," goes the old slogan from books on how businesses should handle complaints. But even when the owner or manager is serious, which I suppose would be naive to believe, it doesn't follow that the customer will be satisfied with the result of his complaint.

But what happens if the customer has a mental illness? What if the business is a hospital or a mental health center or a psychiatrist's office? I don't have to guess.

At NAMI meetings, in conversations with my son, in interviews with other folk with the disability, I've heard of clients being kept waiting more than two hours outside a doctor or counselor's office. I've heard of a case manager who was handling a client's finances refusing to advance the person money for food or gas, explaining that the client needed to learn to be responsible. Then there are stories of doctors turning an out-

standing bill over to a collection agency. I know of a
hospital ER staff declining to evaluate an extremely agi-
tated person for suicide risk until they produced
evidence of insurance.

Was the person with a mental illness justified to feel
they'd been treated badly?

Not always. Even if the complaint doesn't hold
water, I don't believe somebody at the hospital or the
doctor's office or the mental health center is the best
person to handle the complaint. Let's say you're not the
person in the organization the complaint is directed at.
Say you're the supervisor of case managers. You're not
likely to persuade the person making the complaint
that you're impartial.

I should mention this. In my city, and in many
others across the country, if it's a private business, the
Better Business Bureau will step in to mediate a
customer's complaint.

When the complainant has a mental illness, it
becomes a special case. It's common for such people to
feel discounted, put down by other people. They may
not attend to their appearance or hygiene as they
might. Over the years of battling the illness, they may
not have developed good skills at communication. They
may be poor listeners, become impatient, even strike
out verbally. They may tend to be suspicious of others,
distrusting the good will of the person providing a
service.

The role of ombudsman isn't unheard of in mental
health. In Minnesota, the people at the ombudsman's
office in St. Paul represent people who feel they're
victims of "delay, injustice or the impersonal delivery of
services."

In Montana, the state provides the same kind of advocacy for those with a mental illness. Here in Indiana, the state contracts with Mental Health America to provide an ombudsman at the state level and funds an ombudsman at MHA chapters around the state. Monroe County's ombudsman in Bloomington, home of Indiana University, does what the official in most counties does—connects people with the right services and acts as a mediator to resolve conflicts between an individual with the mental illness and some agency or institution.

Who can be an ombudsman? It's obvious that the person must be a good listener and somebody who can state clearly the point of view of each party to the dispute. Beyond this, I would count it a plus if the ombudsman has a knack for coming up with creative solutions—a Solomon at problem solving. Some folk are a natural. But the skills can be learned. For that reason, I argue the candidate for such a position undergoes formal training in mediation.

Any support group such as NAMI can seek funding from local or state government to create an ombudsman's office. Any agency, including a mental health center, can set aside funds for that purpose as well. One thing that's most critical: No matter who creates the position, the ombudsman can't directly be dependent on their income from any group that might be involved in a dispute.

I think everybody wins with an ombudsman. Every time that person succeeds at helping to resolve a conflict, it gives the institution or agency new credibility with people who are being served. When the ombudsman intervenes, it's always a good chance for the directors and managers to learn how to do a better job. It can even lead to reform in, say, a hospital psychiatric ward or the case manager program of a mental health center or the treatment of people in a group home.

But the person with the complaint gains most of all. The illness can rob such people of belief in the good will of others. It can reinforce the person's lack of a sense of self-worth. It can reinforce expectations of always being ill-treated. An ombudsman can help change all that. If the ombudsman succeeds in resolving a complaint, it gives the person standing. It shows that he or she is right to expect fair treatment. A fair, just settlement of the complaint confers status. It nurtures self-worth.

In 1809, the Swedish parliament created the first ombudsman's office. I bet none of those lawmakers dreamed that appointing an agent for ordinary citizens to intercede on their behalf could make such a difference in people's lives 200 years later. But the jury's been out and back. The verdict's in. The ombudsman can set things right. To the mentally ill, for whom so much is wrong, getting a complaint settled fairly would feel like a nice change.

Part VI
The Reforms

Sometimes, the greatest challenge of all is to fix the things that need it in programs that already exist. Or scrap them.

32. Screen Educational Programs

I wondered what kind of film on suicide the lady from the mental health association could show to a group of tenth-graders in their health class.

The lights dimmed. On the screen came one of those seemingly ubiquitous, motivational speakers. In the film, he was speaking to a gym filled with high-schoolers. He spoke the kids' language. Threw in slang. Seemed buddy-buddy. Up flashed photographs of a few kids who had committed suicide. Mr. Charisma then reminded us of how bad their parents must have felt.

He went on to tell the kids that suicide was the easy way out, the coward's way of dealing with problems. Again, he reminded his audience of how taking one's own life was so thoughtless of the feelings of others.

The film left me angry and depressed. The plan was for me to attend the health classes for the rest of the day. That meant sitting through that film four times more. I politely excused myself at the end of that first class.

I was sure that the lady from the mental health association had previewed the film and had decided that the speaker's admonitions were the kind of message the kids needed to hear. Who was I to tell her that I had found the speaker giving kids exactly the wrong message? Who was I to bring up the studies conducted by researchers at Columbia University?

As I recall, at the beginning of the film, viewers were told that it had the seal of approval by some national educational organization. That didn't spare students in that suburban school from a pointless and counterproductive scolding about suicide.

You can go to your public library. You can search the internet. You can check out web sites of support groups. You can find videos, DVDs, books, workbooks, slides and brochures on mental illness. Drug companies put out reams of literature. So do the professional organizations that represent the psychologists, the psychiatrists and social workers. The federal Center for Disease Control (CDC) is yet another source. And SAMHSA, another federal agency, offers even more. It is a dizzying array of material. Some of it is authoritative and useful. Some isn't. Some is just plain dangerous.

I've seen DVDs on mental illnesses that contain misinformation. I've found books that tell you mental illness is a conspiracy invented by self-serving practitioners. I've gone to lectures on mental illness in which the speaker appeared to be overstating where the science on causes is today. I've also attended conferences where the researchers presented general audiences with such technical facts that I doubted most people got anything out of the lectures.

I have to believe that only the unscrupulous intend to mislead, whether by a video, book or speech. I take as a given the good will of others here. But consider this. When school corporations decide on new textbooks, every district in the country sets up a committee, usually including parents as well as educators, to review the texts that are being considered. In some districts, experts from area universities are invited to join the review committees.

I'm proposing that communities create such a group to screen materials on mental illness. The group not only would review the book or DVD for facts. It would also assess if it's being presented well. You want your material to avoid jargon and hysteria. You want it to be effective for its intended audience.

So often I've heard people complain about the media. To be sure, films, TV and newspapers often foster the stereotypes about mental illness. But it's not just the mass media that wrongly portray mental illness. Those who work and advocate within the mental health system can fall into the same trap.

Any number of groups in a community could take the lead in screening educational tools and speakers on mental illness. In one town, it might be the community mental health center. In another it could be the local NAMI chapter. In still another, a group of professionals could take on the responsibility.

You'd want any committee to include family members, those people with the illness and a psychiatrist or psychologist. This committee should also include a respected educator, somebody who has a clear idea of when films or books likely click with an audience.

There is no doubt about it. The guy in the film I saw that day with 20 or so tenth-graders was a terrific speaker. He knew how to connect with kids. This explained why he could make a living out of traveling around the country talking to assemblies of high school students. Indeed, a school principal will invite such a speaker because the very thought of a student's suicide is so terrible to most of us. Yet this speaker made it glamorous, an act that would get everybody's attention, an alternative to a young person's misery.

There are lots of choices for speakers, books and videos. Schools, churches, civic groups, social agencies

—each one could use help in sorting out the good from the bad. This isn't a matter of deciding which TV show to watch tonight. It's a matter of getting the real story of mental illness out. Make it your community's job.

33. Train Community Leaders

I can't be too critical of anyone on the subject of mental illness.

For all the years I've spent learning about the issues, there's still so much I don't understand about mental illness. Where do I get off putting down somebody who recites old and discarded myths about the sundry mental disorders?

But the ignorance that remains abroad hurts a lot of people. When it's a judge or a department head in a large corporation or a school principal, what they don't know can ruin somebody's life.

There are a hundred ways anyone can learn the facts about mental illness. That can make all the difference in the world.

Every manager deals with employees who suffer depression. Does the manager tell them to buck up and get over it? Does that manager move to fire the unproductive employee? Or does he or she counsel the employee to get help before the depression deepens and the person is unable to work altogether?

I bet a lot of managers don't know this. But more hours in just about any given business or organization are lost to depression than to heart disease. It can make a whole bunch of difference if the manager grasps this and knows how to deal with the mentally troubled employee.

Knowing something about mental illness makes a big difference for leaders in many fields. Take the courts.

You expect the prosecutor to take the view that the defendant isn't mentally ill but a cold-blooded killer who has to be put away for life or nobody's safe on the streets.

Sometimes, however, even the judge blows it. I've followed cases where the expert testimony established the profound illness of the defendant. On what basis can a graduate of a law school substitute his or her judgment for that of the psychiatrist who not only had his office wall covered with relevant degrees but had spent his career dealing with people's mental illnesses?

I mentioned earlier the case of severely disturbed Joe Corcoran. The death penalty result in that case prompted my visit with the chancellor of the Fort Wayne campus of Indiana University and Purdue University. I proposed we establish a center where people in the community, starting with judges, could learn more about mental illness. Such leaders should hear the latest research. And they should learn from those with a mental illness and their families. I know from our family's experience that this disability is a lot more than a diagnosis and a label.

I include in this important group educators, namely the teachers, principals and others on the front lines with children every day. These people confront mental health issues, but few have the knowledge and the skill to be effective. Like almost every other professional group, I'm pretty sure most educators enter their positions with their heads full of the nonsense that validates the stigma of mental illness.

I don't know of a school of education that requires future teachers to take a course in mental illness. As a board member of the Education Writers Association, having served a couple of years as president, I attended numerous workshops and conferences. Educators and academics proposed most of the topics. During my 10-year tenure, we did not get the first proposal to hear about what schools need to do to address mental illness. So education reporters from all over the country failed to hear of any push to make tackling mental illness a priority in school reform. It's little wonder mental disorders have been missing from the reform agenda.

What a change a few simple things could make if a teacher understood that the child constantly disrupting the class with his chatter might be suffering from a bipolar disorder. Suppose the teacher didn't scold such a child. Instead, suppose the teacher just listened quietly to the child away from the other kids. That would have a better chance than scolding to get the child to settle down. Training teachers and other educators in mental health issues would give them a new way of seeing the disruptive or otherwise troubled child.

Workshops and conferences are among the most familiar ways to introduce such community leaders to some of the fine points of mental illness. Well-run, led by informed speakers, the typical workshop format gives people a chance to ask questions. During the break over lunch, people can discuss their experiences with others attending the sessions. The trouble is, there are no good ways to see how well the new information has changed people's thinking.

I prefer that the experts make their presentations where the community leaders work.

Then, you can schedule follow-up meetings for this group of people. This not only permits evaluation. But the experts can also invite, say, teachers to tell their stories and offer new strategies for dealing with children who present with mental health issues.

With such programs, you're not only asking people to get smarter. You're asking them to change their attitudes and behavior. The new insights on mental illness may conflict with their deeply held values. For example, some judges are so committed to punishing offenders that they refuse to make allowances for mental illness. A few managers may be so much in the habit of dealing with employees in one way that they can't change no matter how hard they try. Some teachers respond impulsively to kids, even when they know better.

These caveats aside, I believe most of us can learn, can change and become good role models in dealing with folk who have a mental illness. Further, I believe most of us sincerely want to treat others, no matter what their problems are, with kindness and justice. So I have hope.

34. Involve Hospital Staff

I met my son at the ER. This was years after the near tragedy when he was a teenager.

This time, they put him on a bed in one of those wards where every aisle looks the same and you're never sure where you are.

This was 15 or so years ago.

He had called, said he was depressed and would I meet him at the hospital. Of course I told him and I zipped across town as quickly as I could.

We waited in our little space, between the curtains, and didn't say much of anything. There was no talk of how the Reds were doing or what Reagan was up to now. We waited. We waited for quite a while.

Somebody stuck his head in to say they'd sent for the social worker at the psychiatric unit next door to come by to do an assessment.

Couldn't a nurse or ER doctor assess suicide risk? Surely they have the training. We wouldn't have to wait so long. It seemed pretty quiet in the ER that evening.

For years, I'd heard police officers complain that anytime they took a psychiatric patient to the ER, they might have to wait hours for an assessment and a decision of whether or not to admit the person.

Here's the thing. The training of nurses, doctors and other personnel at a hospital varies widely. Who knows what they know about mental illness? Who knows what their attitudes are about the disability? No matter what the person's complaint, admission practices vary widely, too. In my fortunately few trips to an ER, I've encountered this variation in my own community.

Since the city adopted the Crisis Intervention Team to handle a mental health crisis, I've heard officers report that they much prefer dealing with the ER staff at one hospital rather than at another.

Once you move to the psychiatric unit, you enter an altogether different world. I think of it as a cross between a high school and a nursing home. A big part of it for the staff is managing the patients. Like a high school, it's a place that's big on rules. And like a nursing home, the staff is expected to be caring and to dispense medications.

It takes a special person to balance all this and not leave the patient feeling worse than when he or she was admitted. As a rule, the pay is not good. So you typically get a lot of turnover. Again, like the ER staff, you don't know whether the psychiatric ward's staff training was any good. I've had directors of such units admit staff training was woefully inadequate, and this was despite national and state standards. No wonder that you often get a poor outcome with hospital staff.

What does the staff know about the latest anti-psychotic drugs, the side effects, the warning signs of suicide risk?

But I think you can be reasonably certain that the staff throughout the hospital know even less about the psychiatric patient. Without a doubt, that patient is just as likely to end up in a surgical ward or the cardiac care unit for treatment as in a psychiatric ward.

During one of his hospitalizations, my son called to complain that the staff in the psychiatric ward weren't treating him as an equal. He felt discounted and demeaned. My guess was that the staff had no clue John saw things this way.

In my adult life, I had several surgeries. I've visited countless others in a hospital. You're always treated more or less as a child or a feeble elderly person. That's what you expect. You go home grateful for the superior care, nevertheless complaining about the bill. That's your experience when you don't have a mental illness. That's being in the hospital if you don't already feel ashamed, inadequate, inferior. For a person with a

psychiatric disability, going to the hospital, no matter
the reason, can merely reinforce those feelings, which
so hinder recovery.

This is where I'd like to see communities step in.
Goodness knows I don't want them to tell hospital
administrators how to run their hospital but to offer
understanding and insight into the disability for both
trainees and current staff.

Under NAMI's sponsorship, my son John gives talks
to student nurses about mental illness. The feedback
he gets from these hour-long sessions shows he's really
opened the students' eyes. This NAMI program is an
excellent model for training anyone working with
mentally ill persons in a hospital, no matter what ward
they are in.

Many religious groups require their clergy to
perform a stint as a chaplain in a hospital before the
being ordained. It's called CPE or Clinical Pastoral Education. This is when clergy can be introduced to psychiatric patients, which can only help them become better
ministers to those congregation members battling
mental health problems. For those other hospital staff,
the importance of understanding this disability may be
just as important as it is for clergy.

It should be simple to find out what your local
hospital does to educate staff about mental illness and
how to deal with those who suffer any of the mental
disorders. Then your NAMI chapter or community
mental health center can design a program. In our
community, we have a ready-made place where hospital
staff and those in training can meet folk with a mental
illness and get to know them not as stereotypes but as

individuals. That's the Carriage House, our clubhouse rehabilitation center that I described earlier.

An outside group can provide to hospital staff an important supplement to what a hospital already does to meet the challenge that treating people with mental illness presents. The goal is to send patients home better off than when they were admitted. It could happen a lot more often than it does.

35. Include Clergy

It was the early 1960s. Floyd Heine, a clinical psychologist, was leading our pastoral counseling class. He was a tall fellow, with dark, wavy hair, suit always rumpled. Never really seeming to focus on a particular student, his eyes would dart nervously through his horn-rimmed glasses. That day he was telling us young seminary students a funny story about two giants in psychology of that era, Carl F. Rogers and Rollo May, who were duck hunting together.

As I recall the story, both men fired at the same time at a duck who was quickly gaining altitude. Well as luck would have it, the duck dropped near the blind. Both men started toward their prize. May, mocking Rogers' nondirective therapeutic technique, said, "Oh, you feel this is your duck?" I gathered these psychologists had a good laugh.

In those days, getting young ministers just to be empathetic instead of judgmental probably was the most realistic goal of such a counseling class. Oh, you got a smattering of an introduction to schizophrenia and manic depression in an abnormal psychology class. But probing much into major mental illness, well, that was for the psychiatrists. I just speak for my own training: the counseling class didn't touch the big stuff.

Today, as I mentioned earlier, most clergy are expected to complete weeks of training at a hospital in CPE, or clinical pastoral education. Still, even when these students encounter folks with mental illness, it's likely to be in an extreme form and in a psychiatric ward, as unnatural a setting as you can imagine. No wonder so many members of the clergy have told me they don't feel prepared to counsel persons struggling with clinical depression or anxiety attacks. In 1972, my own, Harvard educated minister visited me in the hospital during my siege of depression.

"I just don't how to help Larry," Glen confessed to my wife.

There are ways to change that.

A few years ago, the Fort Wayne NAMI, the family support group, decided to sponsor a conference just for clergy. Protestants, Catholics, liberal and conservative would be invited. The idea for such a gathering didn't come out of the blue.

I recall a NAMI meeting one Tuesday evening when several family members related stories of how their priest or minister refused to visit their loved one in the hospital, or said cruel and ignorant things to a church member who was battling a mental illness. One young woman spoke up and told of how, at her mother's suggestion, she had gone to the church elders. They decided she was possessed of demons and proposed an exorcism. The visit with the elders left this young woman shaken. More than anything else we heard that evening, her story persuaded the group of the need for a conference.

I think that even those of us who organized the gathering were surprised at the turnout of several hundred members of the clergy. Clearly, these ministers and priests felt their own inadequacy to deal with members of their congregations who were hurting so much with severe mental health issues. We invited a cross-section of speakers for the day-long event: a psychiatrist, a minister who had dealt with a mentally ill brother for years, a therapist trained as a minister, a person with the disability and a family member. Reviews of the conference were highly positive. The criticism: Several members said they wished they'd had two days, rather than just one. That's all the NAMI folk needed to hear. They sponsored two more such conferences during the following two years.

Any hospital, mental health center or religious group could put on a workshop and invite all the clergy in the area. It could be a regular event. The ideal would be for sponsorship to rotate. That gives those attending the conference a better idea of what the resources in the community are and how to tap into them.

What does a member of the clergy need to know about mental illness? They probably don't need a lot of detail on brain chemistry or the theories on causes. But they must understand that the illness has a powerful physical component that makes all the patient's efforts to overcome seem so fruitless.

The clergy need to learn something about the latest treatments and what's effective and with what kinds of patients. They need be able to make an educated guess about the diagnosis and to know when it's beyond their expertise. The clergy need to understand how important it is for the family to support that person. It's highly likely that the family is going through some grieving over their loved one's inability to work and otherwise be happy and productive. A minister's counsel here can be extremely helpful.

However, the hardest thing is for the minister to develop the skills in talking with and ministering to somebody with a mental illness. I doubt if he or she can learn this from listening to a lecture at a workshop. My proposal is for NAMI or other local groups to create a hands-on training workshop.

I have to believe that most clergy try to treat and respect each person as an individual. That's fundamental to the teaching of all the great religions. The illness is not the person. But it can make the person seem unlovely, unlovable.

Yes, the skills are important. The empathy is important. So is knowing this isn't a demon but biology and personality. There's much more. What the members of the clergy offer can be their ability to see past the illness and see the spark of the divine. We've got to be sure to include the clergy in the healing.

36. Include the Doctors

The report from the researchers didn't surprise me.

Our suicide prevention subcommittee raised the money and brought up two researchers to Fort Wayne from Indiana University's School of Medicine in Indianapolis.

Over a couple of days, the pair conducted focus groups with about 25 family doctors in our community. They felt it was a representative sample.

How good are local doctors at diagnosing people at risk of suicide? And how connected are they to the professionals in the mental health system? It's critical to get answers. Here's why. It's family doctors, not mental health professionals, who treat the vast majority of persons with a mental illness.

No surprise at the results, as I said.

Survey after survey has found that family doctors miss the diagnosis of a mental illness about half the time. That's a national average. During my visit at the University of Michigan Depression Center, Director John Greden reminded me of that research. He went on to mention that of the diagnoses the doctors got right, they got the treatment wrong in another half of their patients. The doctors know all this. It's often featured in their medical journals.

In the report on the Fort Wayne doctors, most felt confident of their ability to quickly diagnose a person who was depressed and possibly at risk of suicide. Yet their comments to the I.U. researchers didn't give me much confidence. Several speculated that the reason a patient was depressed was that he or she had made poor choices. Nobody mentioned stress. Nobody said anything about brain chemistry. And nobody talked of a genetic bent toward mental illness.

Further disappointing, the doctors made no mention of seeing a patient with bipolar disorder, which isn't that uncommon. Now if the patient a doctor treats for depression in fact suffers from bipolar disorder, the medication likely will be wrong, perhaps even aggravating the person's disability.

Moreover, these family doctors didn't exhibit much knowledge of the community's resources for further treatment. To be sure, they all made occasional referrals to a psychiatrist. Clearly, there is a disconnect.

That was emphatically reinforced when the I.U. researchers met at a later time with the psychiatrists and other mental health professionals. Most people in this group said they had little direct contact with family doctors. At the same time, they expressed a strong interest in working more with those general practice counterparts.

I'm sure the family doctors are painfully aware that many of their patients have developed a mental illness. They're not indifferent to these patients' needs for treatment. But a family doctor has all too many patients. It's not realistic to expect this overworked practitioner to spend half an hour or so with one patient to ferret out a complicated mental health problem. Time won't allow it. The limited reimbursement from insurance companies and federal programs would make such a lengthy office call a financial sacrifice.

Doctors can use screening tools. Perhaps they can even add a few items on depression to the questionnaire the patient is already filling out in the waiting room. That likely would lead to a more accurate diagnosis than basing it on a brief interview. But if you're going to be successful in treating somebody with chronic depression, for example, you've got to do a great deal more than getting the diagnosis and medication right. Somebody—a social worker, a psychologist, a nurse practitioner—needs to monitor the patient who suffers from such a stubborn and capricious illness.

The University of Michigan's Depression Center has been piloting a promising alternative with family doctors in Flint, Michigan. The doctor heading this program takes as a given that others like himself must cope with too many patients to provide the case management that a person with a mental illness requires. So the center has raised the funds to provide a mental health specialist in some of the doctors' offices. Dr. Mike Klinkman, himself a family doctor on the Depression Center staff, told me how this program works. This specialist consults with the doctor to be sure the patient is on the right medication. And, acting on behalf of the doctor, he or she checks regularly in on the patient to see how things are going, whether there's a need to change the medications and just to maintain that link. The person also helps the patient get appointments with a psychiatrist or therapist.

So here's one approach any community could launch. You don't have to be connected to a major research and treatment institution, such as the University of Michigan's Depression Center. Of course, you're looking here at a major fund-raising effort. That can be tougher than the U of M program, which already enjoys an outstanding national reputation as a medical center. What works in Flint, Michigan, might not work in Dallas, Texas, or Fort Wayne, Indiana, but this doesn't matter.

You start addressing any shortcoming in any system by getting the views and the advice of people who run that system. You won't change a thing without enlisting their support anyway. In the case of mental illness, every area in the country has a community mental health center in the region. Many have NAMI chapters and a Mental Health Association, known these days as Mental Health America. Any college or university can organize a forum and invite local and outside speakers. Any medical center or clinic can do the same. And I can guarantee you this. There is in every community at least one financially well off family with a son or daughter, father or mother who has a mental illness, who perhaps even committed suicide. For many people, a family tragedy can become the inspiration to take on mental illness as a mission.

I can't think of anything that would make a bigger difference for those who suffer from a mental illness than to enlist family doctors. They might well need further education, which can be offered informally. How do they talk to patients about depression and anxiety? Do they lecture the patient as they might about overweight or smoking? Or do they accept the person's complaints in a matter-of-fact fashion? Do they tell them it's perfectly natural for anyone to have such feelings? Do these doctors help the patient accept the challenge of this illness? I can't imagine what professionals could be better suited to help a community overcome the stigma of mental illness.

Yes, we want all our doctors to do no harm. That's their sacred oath. But when it comes to mental illness, the family doctors can do a lot of good, too.

37. Invent a New System

If I were to make the case that the mental health system is broken, I'd simply mention what everybody knows:

We only help a fraction of those who need it.

Here are 20 ideas for getting to work on a new system:

1. Create a coordinating council. We have one in Fort Wayne that includes a judge, the mental health center director, heads of various agencies, activists, a psychiatrist. And there is one journalist, me.

2. Ask the council to imagine what a new system would look like, one that reaches everyone in need. What would be different? What of the old system would we keep?

3. Be sure to involve consumers, those persons battling mental illness every day. They know more about what's lacking now than anybody else. They are the authorities on the short-comings, the injustices, the screw-ups.

4. Inventory current services. What does your community offer now? How many people are served over the year? What measures do you use to evaluate outcomes?

5. Identify the gaps. Do the services reach all populations? Minorities? The elderly? What are the numbers?

6. Decide on your greatest need. This can tell you when and where to start with reform.

7. Determine whether persons with addictions are getting mental health treatment or drug and alcohol rehabilitation only. Mental illness can exhibit many faces. One can be addiction.

8. Find out how other communities address the gaps in services and what innovations in treatment they've developed.

9. Raise money to pay a director of that coordinating council.

10. Get academic researchers to look at how police handle persons with a mental illness.

11. Ask the researchers to see whether people released from the hospital are better off than before they were admitted.

12. Set goals. These could be: 10 more psychiatric beds in hospitals; a conference for local therapists; a proposal for more funding for the state division of mental health from the legislature. Be sure consumers of mental health services give input and agree to the goals.

13. Compare what your community offers with what the professional organizations recommend. Do you have enough child psychiatrists? A sufficient number of case managers?

14. Involve community leaders in your planning. Involve the mayor, the president of the city council, the school superintendent.

15. Look ahead. Come up with a five-year plan. Decide what to accomplish and when.

16. Get commitments from everyone at the coordinating council table. What is each one willing to do? How will this get done? You want to meet regularly and hear reports from committees. People have to be accountable. Such work is too important to let anybody slack off.

17. Decide whether the group makes decision by majority or consensus. Make this determination at the formation of your coordinating council.

18. Put your mission in writing. Make it memorable. This will keep your group focused and remind you of why you're spending time and effort on the project.

19. Have each member tell what he, she or the agency does. People in the system often know little about the work of the other parts of the system.

20. Invite the news media to meetings. It's the best way of creating understanding of your goals in the community. Without community support, you'll fail. With it, you'll succeed.

One way or another, one time or another, we're all touched by mental illness. We're touched in our families, in our schools, in the workplace, in our churches, in our neighborhoods. The help and healing that's called for is, well, everyone's business.

Recommended Reading

Redfield, K. (1995). *An unquiet mind: A memoir of moods and madness.* New York: Alfred A. Knopf Inc..

Memoir from a leading researcher of her own battle with bipolar disorder. Enlightening and compelling account.

Barber, C. (2008). *Comfortably Numb: How psychiatry is medicating a nation.* New York: Pantheon.

A critical look at the use of antidepressants for mild mental health problems, favors instead cognitive behavior therapy.

Earley, P. (2006). *Crazy: A father's search through america's mental health madness.* New York: GP Putman's Sons Penguin Group.

Finalist for the Pulitzer Prize. Veteran journalist chronicles how his mentally ill son got caught up in the justice system and intersperses that with the story of the mistreatment of the mentally ill in the Miami system.

Hallowell, E. & Ratey, J. (1995). *Driven to distraction: Recognizing and coping with attention deficit disorder from childhood through adulthood.* New York: Touchstone.

The bible on attention deficit disorder, a condition sometimes confused with a childhood onset of bipolar disorder.

APA (2000). *Diagnostic and Statistical Manual of Mental Disorders 4th Ed. Text Revision (DSM-IV-TR)* Arlington VA: APA Press.

Indispensable and authoritative on the current science in mental illness.

Fisher, R. & Ury, W. (2000) *Getting to yes: Negotiating agreement without giving in, 2nd. Ed.* Harvard Negotiation Project. New York: Penguin Books.

Excellent resource for strategies advocates for mental health can use in almost any situation.

Grollman E. & Malikow, M. (1999) *Living when a young friend commits suicide.* Boston: Beacon Press.

These grief counselors offer practical guidance for living through tragedy.

Manamy, J. (2006). *Living well with depression and bipolar disorder.* New York: Collins.

Highly readable and thorough treatment of these most common psychiatric disabilities.

Whitaker, R. (2002). *Mad in america: Bad science, bad medicine, and the enduring mistreatment of the mentally ill.* Cambridge: Perseus Publications.

A depressing but insightful history of the treatment of the mentally ill in this country. Critical of the psychiatric profession and drug companies.

US Dept of HHS (2001) *National strategy for suicide prevention.* Rockville MD.

Comprehensive model for community action.

Jamison, K.R. (1999). *Night falls fast: Understanding suicide.* New York: Vintage Books.

Compelling read on suicide by the well-known researcher who has tried it.

Rogers, C. (1961) *On becoming a person.* Boston: Houghton Mifflin Co.

Not just a classic for therapists. This book can help anyone searching for a way to deal with people struggling with their own mental demons.

Torrey, E. (2006) *Surviving schizophrenia: A manual for families, consumers, and providers.* New York: Collins.

Standard text for families and advocates.

Greden, J. *Treatment of recurrent depression. review of psychiatriy* Vol. 201. American Psychiatric Publishing Inc. Washington DC.

Professional yet readable collection of essays on depression that resists treatment.

Internet Resources

(In alphabetical order)

AAPC.org. Web site for the American Association of Pastoral Counselors.

Bazelon.org. Washington, D.C. group that advocates for the legal rights of persons with a mental illness.

Bipolaradvantage.com Practical help for persons with this disability.

Bipolarworld.com. More resources on bipolar disorder.

Borderlinedisorder.org. Help for this hard-to-treat psychiatric disorder.

Drugs.com. Good resource on psychiatric medications.

EmotionsAnonymous.org. Follows a 12-step program similar to AA toward recovery.

ICCD.org. Site of the International Center for Clubhouse Development, the group that promotes and supports the clubhouse rehabilitation model.

InternetMentalHealth.com. Attractive site, wide-ranging resource.

MentalHealthAmerica.org. Formerly the National Mental Health Association, this granddaddy of advocacy groups promotes education, research and support through its hundreds of local chapters.

MentalHealthRecovery.com. Upbeat site, features WRAP, which allows persons with the disability to make plans for any crisis, including hospitalization.

Mindfreedom.org. Group's site with current data on advocacy for mental health consumer rights.

NationalMentalHealthInformationCenter.org. From the U.S. Department of Health and Human Services. Very comprehensive resource.

NAMI.org. Site for the National Alliance on Mental Illness, which represents more than a quarter of a million family members. Comprehensive help for families and consumers.

NIMH.nih.gov. Site for the National Institute of Mental Health, whose primary role is to conduct research on mental health issues.

About the Author

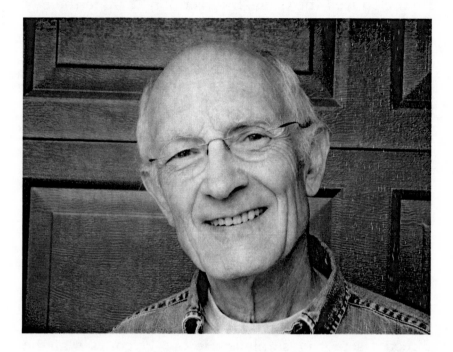

For more than a quarter century, Larry Hayes served as the editorial page editor of the Fort Wayne Journal Gazette. Here, he draws on his years of writing about mental illness and his own personal experience. What he presents is a call to action for entire communities. The book is replete with scores of practical answers to bringing those who suffer out of the shadows and into the mainstream. With real solutions and not just theories, he demonstrates why he has won more than 50 state and national awards for editorials and columns. In 1986, he was finalist for the Pulitzer Prize in recognition of his editorials challenging his city to fully desegregate its schools.

Through editorials and personal urging, Hayes was instrumental in Indiana's victorious fight to win parity of health insurance for persons with a mental illness. He introduced the Crisis Intervention Team to the city to help police better respond to a mental health crisis. He won support for the creation of the Suicide Prevention Council, and a countywide Mental Health Coordinating Council. He played a key role in building public support for the Carriage House, a highly acclaimed rehabilitation center. He successfully lobbied Indiana University Purdue University, Fort Wayne to create the Institute for Behavior Studies, one of the first such programs in the country. His persistent advocacy persuaded the state to transfer an emotionally disturbed 14-year-old girl from the Indiana Women's Prison to a juvenile treatment center.

Hayes holds degrees in theology and education. He has served churches as a student minister. Just out of graduate school, he taught high school English and directed senior class plays. He taught courses at the Indiana University Purdue University in writing, journalism and peace studies. He's written for numerous professional publications. His work also has appeared in *The Wall Street Journal*, *The New York Times*, *Christian Science Monitor* and *The Nation*. He retired in 2000 to write books, starting with *Monday I'll Save the World*, memoir of the heartland journalist, published in 2004.

He serves on numerous boards and committees, living in Fort Wayne with his wife, Dr. Toni Kring, a retired educator. He has two children, Robyn, a Spanish teacher and mother to two teenage girls, and John, an advocate for the mentally ill who suffers from bipolar disorder.

Index

CPSIA information can be obtained at www.ICGtesting.com
Printed in the USA
LVOW062115180812

294919LV00003B/102/P